Managing Health Programs and Projects

Managing Health Programs and Projects

Beaufort B. Longest, Jr.

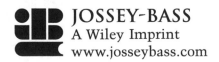

JOSSEY-BASS
A Wiley Imprint
www.josseybass.com

Published by Jossey-Bass
A Wiley Imprint
989 Market Street, San Francisco, CA 94103-1741   www.josseybass.com

This publication is designed to provide accurate and authoritative information in regard to the subject matter covered. It is sold with the understanding that the publisher is not engaged in rendering professional services. If professional advice or other expert assistance is required, the services of a competent professional person should be sought.

Extract on p. 264 is reprinted with permission from *Crossing the Quality Chasm: A New Health System for the 21st Century* by the National Academy of Sciences, courtesy of the National Academies Press, Washington, D.C.

Jossey-Bass books and products are available through most bookstores. To contact Jossey-Bass directly, call our Customer Care Department within the U.S. at 800-956-7739 or outside the U.S. at 317-572-3986, or fax to 317-572-4002.

Jossey-Bass also publishes its books in a variety of electronic formats. Some content that appears in print may not be available in electronic books.

Library of Congress Cataloging-in-Publication Data
Longest, Beaufort B., Jr.
  Managing health programs and projects / Beaufort B. Longest, Jr.—1st ed.
       p.; cm.
  "A Wiley Imprint."
  Includes bibliographical references and index.
  ISBN 0-7879-7185-5 (alk. paper)
 1. Public health administration. 2. Organizational change.
  [DNLM: 1. Health Services Administration. 2. Organizational Innovation.
3. Total Quality Management. W 84.1 L852m 2004] I. Title.
  RA427.L64 2004
  610'.685—dc22

                                                    2004007486

Printed in the United States of America
FIRST EDITION
HB Printing 10 9 8 7 6 5 4 3 2

CONTENTS

FIGURES, TABLES, AND EXHIBITS

Figures

Tables

Exhibit

For Carolyn

Oh, the comfort–the inexpressible comfort of feeling safe with a person–having neither to weigh thoughts nor measure words, but pouring them all right out, just as they are, chaff and grain together; certain that a faithful hand will take and sift them, keep what is worth keeping, and then with the breath of kindness blow the rest away.

Dinah Mulock Craik
A Life for a Life, 1859

PREFACE

This book is about managing health programs and projects. I provide information drawn from a number of areas of management research and literature with the intent of helping the reader develop an evidence-based approach to the practice of management in health programs and projects. A focused reader will take away a solid overview of the current best practices in management that apply to managing health programs and projects.

I think it is important to focus on managing at the level of programs and projects because these are the mechanisms through which a great many health services are organized and provided in both the public health and private health sectors. For example, at the prevention end of the health services spectrum, people receive information about safe sex practices through health education programs, or learn how nutrition affects health. At the advanced acute care end of the spectrum of services, individuals receive kidney transplants within the structure of relatively small transplant programs.

A persistent, decades-long trend has created ever larger and more elaborate structures that organize and deliver health services throughout the industrialized world. Evidence of this trend can be seen in the organization charts of major public health agencies(such as California Department of Health Services http://www.dhs.cahwnet.gov/home/organization/), as well as in the size and complexity of large private-sector health care organizations (such as the University of Pittsburgh Medical Center http://www.upmc.com/Overview.htm).

However, within these large and complex structures, public and private health services often are provided directly through health programs and projects. A substantial amount of literature exists about managing large and complex public and private-sector health agencies, organizations, and systems. I have contributed to this literature myself. However, there is relatively little literature about managing at the level of health programs and projects, where so much of the direct delivery of health services increasingly occurs. This book focuses on management in health programs and projects.

The intended audience for this book includes students in public health, health management, and other health professions who wish to prepare themselves for the challenges of managing health programs and projects. Even those who aspire to high-level positions in large agencies, organizations, and systems are likely to begin their management careers at the level of programs and projects. The book is also intended for those in management positions who seek current information about managing.

Health programs and projects are defined as groups of people and other resources formally associated through intentionally designed relationships in order to pursue desired results. Beyond this definition, programs and projects are described as *logic models,* or depictions of how they are supposed to work. A logic model presents a schematic picture of relationships among the inputs or resources available to a program or project, the processes undertaken with the inputs, and the results the program or project is intended to achieve. It is not possible to fully understand a program or project—or to manage it effectively—without first understanding its logic model.

Health programs or projects target any of the determinants of health, such as the physical environments in which people live and work, peoples' behavior, peoples' biology, the social factors that affect people, or health services provided to them. Thus, there is a broad array of health programs and projects. Health programs and projects might focus, for example, on cancer care, nutrition, geriatric care, women's health services, palliative care, health education, migrant worker health care, safe sex practices, cleaning up the physical environment, cardiac rehabilitation, or smoking cessation. The most important distinction between programs and projects is that projects form a subset of programs, distinguished by the fact that projects are time-limited. Projects have predetermined life cycles, while programs are managed as ongoing entities. Otherwise, their management is essentially the same.

In both public and private sectors, health program or project management is defined as the *activities* through which the desired outputs, outcomes, and impact of a program or project are established and pursued through various processes that use human and other resources. This definition of management requires consideration of management work in terms of the activities that make up the work.

All health program and project managers engage in three core activities as they perform management work: *strategizing, designing,* and *leading.* In performing these core activities, managers also engage in other activities that facilitate and support accomplishment of the core activities. These facilitative activities are *decision making, communicating, managing quality,* and *marketing.* The core and facilitative activities that make up management work give this book its structure.

Chapter One, "Management Work," provides an overview of management work in health programs and projects, as well as some key definitions and concepts, all of which serve as a framework for the remainder of the book. The centerpiece of this chapter is Figure 1.4, which depicts the core and facilitative activities of management work.

Chapter Two, "Strategizing the Future," discusses how managers, often with the involvement of others, establish the desired results to be achieved through a program or project and conceptualize the means of accomplishing the goals. This chapter is organized around how managers in an ongoing program or project answer four critical questions:

What is the current situation of our program or project?

In what ways do we want our program or project's situation to change in the future?

How will we move our program or project to the preferred future state?

Are we making acceptable progress toward the desired future state?

Chapter Three, "Designing for Effectiveness," discusses how managers shape two important aspects of their programs and projects. Consideration is given to how managers establish and revise the logic models of their programs and projects. Consideration is also given to how managers establish and revise the *organization designs*–the intentional patterns of relationships among human and other resources–of their programs and projects.

Chapter Four, "Leading to Accomplish Desired Results," defines leading by managers as *influencing* others to understand and agree about what needs to be done in order to achieve the desired results established for a program or project, and facilitating the individual and collective contributions of others to achieving the desired results. As managers seek to influence other participants to behave in contributory ways, they must understand how to help them be motivated to do so. Thus, the relationship between human motivation and success in leading is emphasized.

Chapter Five, "Making Good Management Decisions," focuses on decision making as a pervasive facilitative activity in management work, permeating the core activities of strategizing, designing, and leading, as well as the other facilitative activities of communicating, managing quality, and marketing. Although decision making is defined simply as making a choice from among alternatives, the decision-making process is discussed in terms of seven steps: (1) becoming aware that a decision must be made, whether the decision stems from a problem or an opportunity; (2) defining in as much detail as possible the problem or opportunity; (3) developing relevant alternatives; (4) assessing the alternatives; (5) choosing from among the alternatives; (6) implementing the decision; and (7) evaluating the decision and making necessary follow-up decisions.

Chapter Six, "Communicating for Understanding," discusses a facilitative activity that is both vital to the successful performance of management work and a challenge for managers. Communicating is described as an activity that involves senders. Senders can be individuals, groups, or organizations, conveying ideas, intentions, and information to receivers. Receivers can also be individuals, groups, or organizations. Communication is effective when receivers understand ideas, intentions, or information as senders intend, but several environmental and interpersonal barriers must be overcome to communicate effectively. The communicating activity is discussed as a key to managing relationships with a program or project's internal and external stakeholders.

Chapter Seven, "Managing Quality–Totally," discusses why managers of health programs and projects typically give a high priority to effectively managing the quality of services provided. Not only is quality important to those who receive the services of a program or project, quality is important to participants who work in programs and projects. This chapter stresses that, above all else, managing quality in a program or project requires a systematic approach. Three principles that can guide managers in pursuit of what is called a *total quality* (TQ) approach to managing quality in health programs and projects are presented: patient/customer focus, continuous improvement, and teamwork.

Chapter Eight, "Commercial and Social Marketing," as the title suggests, discusses two important ways managers of health programs and projects can use marketing to facilitate success. The financial or commercial success of many programs and projects is affected by the use of *commercial marketing*. In addition, especially in programs and projects focused on health promotion and education, *social marketing* is used in the provision of services. The so-called 4 Ps of successful commercial marketing strategies are discussed: **p**roduct or service, **p**rice, **p**lace, and **p**romotion. Social marketing is discussed in terms of using elements of commercial marketing to influence the voluntary behavior of individuals and groups of people for their own benefit—and in some instances for the larger society's benefit.

It is convenient for purposes of discussion or description to separate into individual chapters the core and facilitative activities that make up management work. Doing so, however, might incorrectly suggest that the core and facilitative activities are a series of separate activities, perhaps performed in a particular sequence. In practice, managers of health programs and projects engage in these activities as a whole in which the various activities are highly interrelated and interdependent. When managers integrate and perform the activities well, they are more likely to be satisfied with the performance of their programs and projects, and with the results achieved. My main purpose in writing this book, then, is to help managers achieve desired levels of performance in health programs and projects and accomplish the results they seek through those programs and projects.

Acknowledgments

I wish to acknowledge the contributions made by several people to this book and to thank them for their assistance. At the University of Pittsburgh, which has been my professional home for twenty-four years, Linda Kalcevic provided superb editorial support throughout the many drafts. Denise Warfield provided cheerful and helpful secretarial support. Mark Nordenberg, Arthur Levine, Bernard Goldstein, and Judith Lave provided an environment conducive to and supportive of scholarship. At Jossey-Bass, Andy Pasternack saw the potential for this book and has been a partner in its development and publication. I also wish to thank Jessica Egbert, Gigi Mark, and Seth Schwartz for their professional expertise in this project. Most of all, however, I want to thank Carolyn Longest, whose presence in my life has made many things possible—and doing them seem worthwhile.

June 2004   Beaufort B. Longest, Jr.
Pittsburgh, Pennsylvania

THE AUTHOR

Beaufort B. Longest, Jr. is the M. Allen Pond Professor of Health Policy and Management in the Department of Health Policy and Management in the Graduate School of Public Health at the University of Pittsburgh. He also holds a secondary appointment as professor of business administration in the Katz Graduate School of Business, and is director of the University of Pittsburgh's Health Policy Institute.

He received his undergraduate degree from Davidson College and received his M.H.A. and Ph.D. degrees from Georgia State University.

Longest is a fellow of the American College of Healthcare Executives and is a member of the Academy of Management, AcademyHealth, the American Public Health Association, and the Association for Public Policy Analysis and Management. He was elected to membership in both the Beta Gamma Sigma Honor Society in Business and the Delta Omega Honor Society in Public Health.

His research on issues of health policy and management has generated substantial grant support and has led to the publication of numerous peer-reviewed articles. In addition, he has authored or co-authored ten books and twenty-eight chapters in other books. Two of his books, *Managing Health Services Organizations and Systems* and *Health Policymaking in the United States,* are among the most widely used textbooks in graduate health policy and management programs.

Longest consults with health care organizations and systems, universities, associations, and government agencies on health policy and management issues.

Managing Health Programs and Projects

CHAPTER ONE

MANAGEMENT WORK

Health is often pursued through a variety of health programs and projects. For example, when a young adult achieves academic success and starts a promising career after overcoming a drug addiction, an effective treatment program may deserve much of the credit for the turnaround. When a person with type 2 diabetes leads an active and productive life, her health improvements may well be attributed to a program that helps her understand the disease and take an active role in controlling it. When a county health department mounts a project to enroll children in an innovative insurance plan, the impact on those children may be felt throughout a lifetime of better health.

One of the distinguishing characteristics of successful programs and projects is how well their managers perform. This book is about the work these managers do. This chapter provides an overview of management work in health programs and projects, as well as some key definitions and concepts, all of which serve as a framework for the remainder of the book. Management work is described in terms of the core activities–strategizing, designing, and leading–managers undertake in performing this work. After reading this chapter, the reader should be able to do the following:

- Define health, health programs and projects, and management
- Understand the core and facilitative activities of managers' work

- Understand the roles managers play as they do management work
- Appreciate the underlying skills and competencies used by managers in doing management work
- Understand the importance of applying well-developed personal ethical standards in doing management work

As a backdrop for considering management work, it is important to know that three distinct types of work occur in health programs and projects (Charns and Gittell 2000). *Direct work* entails the actual provision of services or creation of products for which a program or project exists. This type of work is done by counselors, nurses, therapists, physicians, health educators, and others who form what Mintzberg (1983) terms the "operating core" of a program or project.

A second type of work done in health programs and projects is *support work.* This work is a necessary and facilitative adjunct to the direct work. In health programs and projects, people performing support work are involved in such activities as fund raising and development, recruiting patients for a clinical trial, providing legal counsel, marketing a program or enhancing public relations for a project, or providing accounting and financial services.

The third type of work done in health programs and projects is *management work*. This work involves establishing—often with the direct participation of others—the results a program or project is intended to achieve and creating the circumstances through which the direct work, aided by support work, can lead to the desired results.

An example will clarify the different types of work. A manager may establish the desired result of a project as enrolling one thousand children in an innovative insurance plan. The act of enrolling children in the plan is the direct work of the project. The manager may also arrange for publicity about the plan to increase awareness and encourage enrollment. The provision of publicity is support work. Establishing the desired result, assigning and training project staff to help parents or guardians enroll children, and arranging for publicity is management work.

As we will see in this chapter, there are two basic ways to assess and study management work. It can be approached in terms of the *activities* managers engage in as they do their work and in terms of the *roles* they play in performing this work. We will examine management work from both perspectives. We will also discuss the *skills* and *competencies* needed to do management work well. Before considering management work, however, it will be useful to define key terms such as *health, health programs and projects,* and *management.*

Health and Health Determinants

The World Health Organization (http://www.who.int.htm) provides a long-standing definition of *health* as the "state of complete physical, mental, and social well-being, and not merely the absence of disease or infirmity" (World Health Organization 1948, p. 100). Another version of this definition views health as a state in which the biological and clinical indicators of organ function are maximized and in which physical, mental, and role functioning in everyday life are also maximized (Brook and McGlynn 1991). The state of health in human beings is a function of many variables, or *health determinants,* as they are often called. The wide variety of determinants means that health programs and projects have an enormous range of possible foci.

Health determinants for individuals or populations include the physical environments in which people live and work; their behaviors; their biology (genetic makeup and the physical and mental health conditions acquired during life); a host of social factors that include economic circumstances, socioeconomic position in society, income distribution, discrimination based on factors such as race/ethnicity, gender, or sexual orientation, and the availability of social networks and social support; and the health services to which they have access (Evans, Barer, and Marmor 1994; Berkman and Kawachi 2000). Health programs and projects can be focused on any of these determinants, as well as on combinations of them.

Health Programs and Projects as Logic Models and as Organizations

The most useful way to get a clear picture of what a program is and does is to think of it as a *theory* (Patton 1997; Weiss 1998) or *hypothesis.* Like all theories, the theory of a program or project is simply a plausible, sensible model of how it is supposed to work (Bickman 1987). The way a program or project is intended to work can be described as a theory or hypothesis by developing a series of *if,* *then* statements about it. For example, a particular program or project can be characterized as follows: *If* resources a, b, and c are assembled; and *then* processed by doing m, n, and o with the resources; and *if* the processing is done well, *then* the results will be x, y, and z. Using its underlying theory or hypothesis as a guideline, any program or project can be described in terms of the inputs available for it to use, the processes it undertakes with the resources, and the results it achieves by processing the resources.

Implicit in the hypothesis or theory of a program or project is its underlying rationale or logic (Renger and Titcomb 2002). In fact, for any program or project, it is possible to draw a logic model of how it is supposed to work (W. K. Kellogg Foundation 2001). A logic model presents a schematic picture of the relationships among the inputs or resources available to a program or project, the processes undertaken with the inputs, and the results the program or project is intended to achieve. Figure 1.1 depicts a basic logic model for a program or project.

This logic model shows how *inputs* and *resources* are *processed* in attempting to accomplish the program or project's desired results in the form of *outputs, outcomes,* and ultimately *impact.* In effect, the logic model provides a road map of how a program or project is intended to work. There is a feedback loop from desired results to inputs and resources and processes indicating that adjustments will be necessary in them in an ongoing program or project. Very importantly, it shows the program or project existing within a larger *external environment.*

The external environment of a program or project includes many variables that can influence its performance. These are illustrated in Figure 1.1 by the arrow that flows from the environment into the program or project's logic model. These external variables include everything from the cultural milieu of the community in which the program or project is undertaken to its physical climate. It also includes economic conditions, the state of health of the population the program or project might serve, housing patterns, demographic patterns, political environment, background and experiences of program participants, media influence, public policies, and the priorities and resources of the larger organization in which a program or project may be embedded.

External variables can influence almost everything about a program or project including whom it seeks to serve, the extent of recipients' needs for the program or project's services, the resources available to the program or project, the quality of its staff and volunteers, how smoothly implementation occurs, and the pace at which results are seen. A program or project cannot be completely separated from its external environment. All programs and projects are affected by and affect their external environments.

The results of a program or project flow out into its external environment. This is shown in Figure 1.1 by the arrow that flows outward into the external environment. This arrow means that the outputs, outcomes, and impact of a program or project flow outward and affect the individuals and populations that it serves. The concept of the logic model of a program or project will be useful throughout this book, beginning with how we think about programs and projects as organizations.

FIGURE 1.1. THE LOGIC MODEL OF A PROGRAM OR PROJECT.

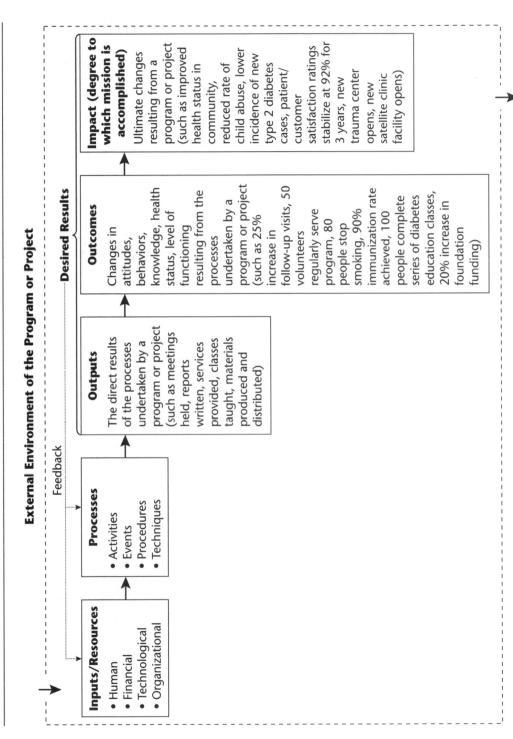

A program or project cannot exist as a theory or hypothesis. Actual programs and projects take the form of groups of people and other resources formally associated with each other through intentionally designed patterns of relationships in order to pursue some pre-established results. That is they exist as *organizations,* albeit rather small ones. Organizations can be very large, involving thousands of participants. Expansive integrated health care systems or state health departments, for example, are large organizations. Even though programs and projects are typically much smaller than such organizations, they meet the definition of organizations. Programs and projects can be defined as groups of people and other resources formally associated with each other through intentionally designed patterns of relationships in order to pursue desired results.

Programs or projects that pertain to any of the determinants of health noted previously are *health programs or projects.* Thus health programs and projects address some aspect of the physical environments in which people live and work, as well as their behaviors, their biology, the social factors that affect them, and health services.

Programs and projects differ in only one major respect, although this difference is important in managing them. Projects are a subset of programs that are time-limited. That is, a project has a *pre-determined life cycle,* and a program has an *indeterminate life cycle.* The duration of a project is scheduled at its beginning, although some run for longer or shorter durations than originally planned because of changing circumstances. Projects have specific beginning and ending points (Frame 2003). Programs have indeterminate life expectancies in that they are expected to go on indefinitely.

Figure 1.2 graphically *depicts a project life cycle.* Assume that the project is intended to conduct diabetes screenings at an annual health fair. The curve reflects the consumption of human, financial, and material resources during the life cycle of the project. A gradual build up of activity during which arrangements are made for the conduct of the screenings precedes the peak of activity when the actual conduct of the screenings occurs. The peak is followed immediately by the project's conclusion and termination.

Examples of *health programs* include those in cancer care, cardiac rehabilitation, data and statistics, geriatrics, health education, home care, palliative care, prevention, promotion, research and development, substance abuse, wellness, and women's health. Less obvious examples of health programs include housing programs, job training, or programs to clean up the physical environment, as well as programs aimed at reducing ignorance, discrimination, or poverty. These less obvious examples are also health programs because they also address one or another health determinant. Appendix A provides a brief description of a health program embedded in the Glendale Adventist Medical Center, Hearts N' Health. Note the ongoing nature of this program reflected in the final paragraph of the description.

FIGURE 1.2. A PROJECT'S LIFE CYCLE.

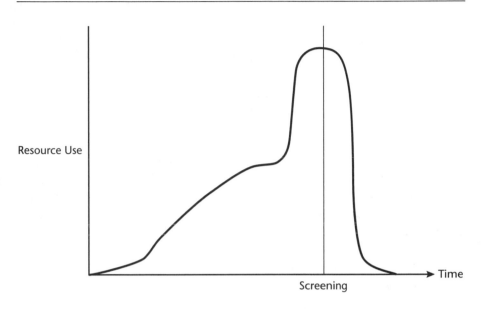

Examples of *health projects* include research or demonstration projects pertaining to a health determinant, as well as projects to promote seat belt use, healthier eating, or safe sex practices. Projects also may be designed to achieve some specific physical or intellectual purpose within a larger program or organization, such as designing and equipping a laboratory, training staff members in a new protocol or how to use some new technology, designing an information system, or developing a strategic plan or a new accounting system. Appendix B provides a brief overview of a project embedded in the Office of Minority Health, U.S. Department of Health and Human Services, to develop a set of national standards for culturally and linguistically appropriate health services. Note that the project terminated with the publication of the standards as reflected in the final paragraph of the overview.

Typically, health programs and projects are embedded within larger organizational settings or homes, such as health departments, hospitals, health plans, nonprofit organizations or agencies, long-term care organizations, or large integrated health systems. Both the program and the project illustrated in Appendices A and B are embedded in larger organizations; one is embedded in a public health agency of the federal government and the other in a private health care organization. It is possible for a program, however, to be freestanding from any other organization, perhaps having its own governing board. When health programs and projects are embedded within larger organizations like departments and other sub-divisions of the larger organizations, it is useful to think of these programs and projects as *organizations within organizations.*

Program and Project Management

Program or project management is defined as the activities through which the desired outputs, outcomes, and impact of a program or project are established and pursued through various processes using human and other resources. Following the basic logic model of a program or project shown in Figure 1.1, it can be seen that managers, often with help from other participants in a program or project, seek to accomplish the following:

- Determine a program or project's desired outputs, outcomes, and impact
- Assemble the necessary inputs and resources to achieve the desired results
- Determine the processes necessary to accomplish the desired results and ensure that the processes are carried out effectively and efficiently
- Do the things noted previously while analyzing variables in the program or project's external environment, assessing their importance and relevance, and responding to them appropriately

In performing management work, managers engage in an interrelated set of *activities* and play a mosaic of interconnected *roles,* both of which are facilitated by possession and use of certain *skills* and *competencies.* The activities in which managers engage as they manage and the roles they play as they perform management work are considered in the next section.

The Work of Managers: Activities and Roles

This book is organized and presented around the *activities* that managers engage in as they manage. Focusing on activities is sometimes called a functional approach to the work of managers. In addition to performing sets of interconnected activities, managers also play certain *roles* as they do management work. In performing activities or playing roles, managers rely upon certain *skills* and *competencies* to do their work well.

This section introduces the activities managers engage in as they perform management work, the roles played in doing this work, and the skills and competencies needed to do this work. Throughout this section and in the more in-depth discussions to follow in the book, the descriptions of and the prescriptions and recommendations about the activities that managers engage in as they perform management work reflect *evidence-based management*. Practicing evidence-based management means that managers, like clinicians practicing evidence-based medicine, base their professional work on empirical evidence from management research (Kovner, Elton, and Billings 2000; Walshe and Rundall 2001).

The Core Activities in Management Work

All health program and project managers engage in three core activities as they perform management work: *strategizing, designing,* and *leading* (Zuckerman and Dowling 1997). In performing these core activities, managers also engage in other activities that facilitate and support accomplishment of the core activities. These facilitative activities are briefly discussed later in this chapter; a subsequent chapter is devoted to each of the activities. The core strategizing, designing, and leading activities of management work are shown in Figure 1.3 and are discussed briefly in the following sections. More detailed discussions of these activities follow in subsequent chapters.

Strategizing. The work that managers do when establishing the outputs, outcomes, and impact desired for their programs and projects—and when conceptualizing the means of accomplishing them—is *strategizing*. Although the relative degree of complexity may vary, managers of all programs and projects engage

FIGURE 1.3. THE CORE ACTIVITIES IN MANAGEMENT WORK.

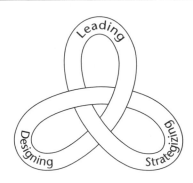

in strategizing activities as part of performing management work. This activity also helps managers adapt their programs and projects to the challenges and opportunities presented by their external environments (Ginter, Swayne, and Duncan 2002).

The aim of strategizing is to achieve an integrated set of direct, support, and management work sufficient to establish and achieve the results envisioned for a program or project. Effective *strategizing* lays the foundation for *designing* effective relationships among people and other resources necessary to achieve desired results. It also provides the blueprint managers use in *leading* others in contributing to their achievement.

There are a number of reasons why strategizing activities are so crucial to the success of health programs and projects. Perhaps none is more important than the simple fact that this activity focuses attention on desired results. Good strategizing yields statements of intended outputs, outcomes, and impact, and conceptualizes the means through which these can be achieved. In this way strategizing contributes to the coordination and integration of the actions of all participants in a program or project toward shared purposes.

Another reason strategizing is important is that it helps offset the pervasive uncertainty that health programs and projects face. When managers think about the future in systematic ways and plan for contingencies that can be imagined or foreseen, they greatly reduce the chances of being caught unprepared. Uncertainty cannot be eliminated, but it can be prepared for through strategizing. Conditions of uncertainty require that programs and projects be adaptable and flexible, which makes strategizing critical.

A third reason strategizing is important is that it enhances efficiency and effectiveness. It facilitates the substitution of coordinated and integrated effort in place of random activity, controlled flow of work in place of uneven flow, and careful decisions in place of snap judgments. As demands increase for programs and projects to be operated efficiently and effectively, the value of strategizing increases.

Finally, strategizing in health programs and projects is important because it facilitates managers' efforts to assess and control results in their programs or projects. Controlling relies upon comparing actual results with some predetermined desired result and taking corrective actions when actual results do not match desired results. Good strategizing yields statements of desired results against which actual results can be compared.

Control techniques are based upon the same basic elements regardless of whether quality, cost, participant or patient and customer satisfaction, or some other variable is being controlled. Controlling, wherever it occurs, involves four steps: (1) establishing standards or desired results, (2) measuring performance, (3) comparing actual results with standards or desired results, and (4) correcting deviations from standards or desired results when they occur.

Designing. *Designing* is the work managers do when establishing the initial logic models of their programs and projects and subsequently reshaping them as circumstances change. Managers are also designing when they establish the intentional patterns of relationships among human and other resources within their programs and projects and when they establish the relationship of the program or project to its external environment, including, when relevant, to the larger organizational homes in which it is embedded.

Guided by the requirements of a program or project's logic model, designing activities permit managers to design and build an organizational structure. This includes assembling the necessary inputs and resources for the program or project. Because human resources are a key resource in all programs and projects, designating individual positions and aggregating or *clustering* these positions into the work groups, teams or other subunits of a program or project is a critical aspect of a manager's designing activity. The number and type of individual positions are typically determined by how a program or project's work is divided and specialized.

In larger programs or projects, designing activity may also include clustering work groups into divisions or other units, as well as determining how the various work groups and clusters of work groups are integrated and coordinated. Depending upon circumstances, designing may also involve relating a program or project to a larger organizational home. For example, a program embedded in a county health department must fit within its larger organizational home. A program manager in such a setting may report to a superior in the larger organizational home.

The pattern of relationships among the human and other resources that results from designing activities is called the *organization design* of a program or project. *Staffing* involves the specific activities of attracting and retaining people to occupy the positions in an organization design, and is thus a vital part of organizing a program or project. In addition to relying upon paid staff, some programs or projects use volunteers.

In practice, organization design proceeds from individual positions through a clustering of positions into work groups, which may serve as subunits of a program or project, or may be the entire program or project. For programs and projects embedded in larger organizations, clustering of work groups forms the organization design of programs, projects, departments, and the larger subdivisions of the organization. Eventually, clustering produces an entire organization and perhaps even a system of inter-connected organizations.

Successful designs in health programs and projects, as well as in larger organizations, depend upon appropriate distributions of *authority* and *responsibility* as the organization is built up through successive rounds of clustering. Authority is the power one derives from a position in an organization design. Responsibility can be thought of as the obligation to execute work, whether it is direct, support, or management work. All participants in programs and projects have responsibilities as a result of their positions. The source of responsibility is one's organizational superior in the organization design. By delegating responsibility to an organizational subordinate, the superior creates a relationship based on mutual obligations between superior and subordinate.

Effective organization designs achieve a balance between authority and responsibility. When responsibility is given to a participant, that person must also be given the necessary authority to make commitments, use resources, and take the actions necessary to fulfill the responsibility.

Depending upon the circumstances of a program or project, a challenge for its design can be the degree of *coordination* required among participants. There is a correlation between the degree to which a program or project's work is divided and the need for attention to coordination among participants. The more differentiated the work is, the more important—and often more difficult—the coordination task is likely to be. For example, in the project to enroll children in an innovative health plan described previously, the work would not be highly differentiated. In contrast, a large program in women's health would involve many different people performing highly differentiated work. Coordination would be more of a challenge in the latter case.

Health programs and projects, and certainly the larger organizations in which many of them are embedded, are often characterized by considerable division of work into a number of professional and technical jobs. The work done in these settings is so often performed by such a variety of workers that very significant coordination problems arise. In addition, the direct, support, and management work in most programs and projects are highly interdependent. This condition of functional interdependence makes achieving coordination an important aspect of the organization design of a program or project.

Another key to successful health program and project organization designs is the inclusion of features that minimize and resolve *conflict* among participants. Individuals participating in programs or projects may perceive missions or objectives differently or may favor various pathways to their fulfillment. Conflict may arise between and among any of the various participants in a program or project, as well as with others outside the program or project.

Conflict involving two or more individuals within a program or project, as well as conflict between a program and its organizational home or other entities, may arise. In fact, both forms of conflict should be anticipated and can be addressed at least partially through organization design. Even such low levels of conflict as those evidenced by some participants disliking other participants or having difficulty in getting along with others can reduce performance in a program or project. Thus, the prevention or resolution of conflict is an important aspect of successful organization designs; effective designs for programs and projects facilitate the management of conflict.

In combination, a program's logic model and its organization design provide a comprehensive snapshot of the program, what it intends to accomplish, and how it intends to accomplish its desired results. The snapshot provides guidance for the third core activity managers engage in as they do management work, leading.

Leading. The work managers do when influencing other participants to contribute to the performance of their programs or projects is *leading*. No matter how well a manager strategizes and designs, a program or project's success also depends upon the manager effectively leading.

In leading the other participants in a program or project, managers seek to instill in them a shared vision of a program or project's logic model, and stimulate determined efforts to make the model work. As leaders, managers focus on the various decisions and actions that affect the entire undertaking, including those intended to ensure the program or project's survival and overall well-being. Leading also requires managers to help participants be *motivated* to contribute to the program or project.

Leading successfully in any setting is a challenge. It is especially so in programs and projects where leaders must satisfy diverse constituencies. Not only must the needs and preferences of a program or project's patients/customers, which themselves are not likely to be homogeneous in their needs and preferences, be taken into account, but so must the needs and preferences of other participants. Only rarely are the needs and preferences of all participants in a program or project in harmony.

As Figure 1.3 illustrates, the core activities of managers are interrelated. Leading is not done in isolation from designing and strategizing. How well managers engage in one of the core activities affects their performance in the others. In addition to these core activities of management work, managers engage in a number of other activities that support and facilitate their performance of the core activities. These facilitative activities are considered next and permit us to create a more complete mosaic of the activities that make up management work.

The Facilitative Activities in Management Work

Managers engage in *decision making* and *communicating* as they perform the core activities of strategizing, designing, and leading. Increasingly, managers of programs and projects also engage in *managing quality* and *marketing* as they seek to assure the success of their programs and projects. Thus, Figure 1.3 can be expanded into a more complete picture of the activities performed in management work. Figure 1.4 shows the *facilitative activities* of decision making, communicating, managing quality, and marketing intertwined with the *core activities* of management work.

Decision Making. Decision-making activities permeate all management work, facilitating a manager's performance of the core activities of strategizing, designing, and leading. Managers make decisions when desired results are established in a program or project's logic model through strategizing, or when alterations are made in a program or project's organization design or logic model. In fact, not only are designs subject to change, but all management work is performed in a dynamic context that requires continual decision making to modify such variables as results, means, tasks, technologies, and people.

Decision making is simply making a choice between two or more alternatives. The myriad decisions that program and project managers face can be divided into two subsets: problem-solving decisions and opportunistic decisions (DuBrin 2003). Problem-solving decisions are made in order to solve existing or anticipated problems. Opportunistic decisions are typically sporadic and arise with opportunities to advance accomplishment of a program or project's intended results.

Communicating. Just as decision-making activities permeate all management work, communicating activities are also ubiquitous in facilitating a manager's performance of the core activities of strategizing, designing, and leading. For example, managers who can effectively articulate and communicate their ideas and

**FIGURE 1.4. THE CORE AND FACILITATIVE
ACTIVITIES IN MANAGEMENT WORK.**

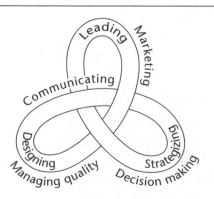

preferences have a distinct advantage in leading a program or project's participants. If participants are to be involved in designing logic models and organization designs, communicating is vital, and if these designs are to be understood by those affected by them, details of the designs must be effectively communicated. Communicating is essential in developing strategies for a program or project and in sharing the strategies with stakeholders inside and outside the program or project.

Communicating involves senders (who can be individuals, groups, or organizations) conveying ideas, intentions, and information to receivers (who can also be individuals, groups, or organizations). Communication is effective when receivers understand ideas, intentions, or information as senders intend. Managers in health programs and projects must be concerned with communication on two levels. They concern themselves extensively with communicating with internal stakeholders in their programs or projects, as well as with communicating between the program or project and other stakeholders in its external environment.

Managing Quality. In successfully managing health programs and projects, managers are heavily involved in *managing quality.* Not only is quality obviously important to those to whom services are provided, it is also important to the people who work in programs and projects. For example, it has been shown that working in environments characterized by efforts to continuously improve quality yields higher levels of satisfaction with work for participants (Berlowitz and others 2003).

In what we will call a *total quality (TQ) approach* in this book, managers are guided by the application of three principles as they seek to manage quality: focusing on the patients/customers of their program or project, striving for continuous improvement, and fostering teamwork (Dean and Bowen 1994). A patient/customer focus means identifying what a program or project's patients/customers need and want and then developing and delivering services that satisfy those needs and wants. Continuous improvement means making a commitment to continuous efforts to examine the processes through which services are provided in search of better ways to provide them. Teamwork is emphasized in a TQ approach because quality is a collective responsibility of all those involved in a program or project.

Marketing. The boundary between a program or project and its external environment is important territory for its manager. Managers use *marketing* to effectively cross these boundaries. The purpose of marketing is to bring about voluntary exchanges of values with others for the purpose of achieving the program or project's objectives. Others in the external environment that can be reached through marketing activities include potential direct patients/customers for a program or project's services, as well as people who can influence patients/customers. Engaging in exchanges with patients and customers is critical to the success of most programs or projects, especially when services for sale are offered.

In addition to patients/customers, successful programs and projects engage in voluntary exchanges with physicians and other health care providers who are in a position to refer patients or consumers, and with insurers and health plans who may permit or limit use of a program or project's services by their subscribers or members. Similarly, voluntary exchanges are made with potential employees and perhaps with donors, volunteers, and organizations in which a program or project is embedded. All of these exchanges are supported and facilitated through marketing.

It is important to stress the interdependence among the full set of activities shown in Figure 1.4, including the core activities of management work (strategizing, designing, and leading) and the facilitative activities of decision making, communicating, managing quality, and marketing. Although it is convenient to separate activities for purposes of discussion or description, the danger in doing so is that it may seem that managing is a series of separate activities, perhaps performed in a particular sequence. In practice, managers do not perform the activities noted earlier separately—and certainly not in a fixed sequence.

The mosaic of core and facilitative activities that managers engage in as they do management work as shown in Figure 1.4 guides the outline for the remaining chapters of this book as follows:

Chapter Two	Strategizing the Future
Chapter Three	Designing for Effectiveness
Chapter Four	Leading to Accomplish Desired Results
Chapter Five	Making Good Management Decisions
Chapter Six	Communicating for Understanding
Chapter Seven	Managing Quality—Totally
Chapter Eight	Commercial and Social Marketing

As subsequent chapters are read, it may be useful from time to time to revisit Figure 1.4 to review how the activities being described fit together into the mosaic of activities that make up management work. Before examining the activities that make up management work in detail, however, it will be useful to consider this work from another vantage point—the roles managers play as they perform management work.

Roles Played by Managers: The Mintzberg Model

Although it was conducted decades ago and did not focus specifically on managers of health programs or projects, an important study of management work has direct applicability to considering the work of managers in programs and projects. Henry Mintzberg (1973; 1975) observed a sample of managers over a period of time, recorded and analyzed what they did, and concluded that management work can be described meaningfully in terms of three categories of interrelated roles that all managers play. Thus, another way to examine the work of managers is to think about the different roles they play.

Roles are the typical or customary sets of behaviors that accompany particular positions. Teachers play identifiable roles in schools, quarterbacks play defined roles on football teams, and managers play roles as they perform management work. Mintzberg concluded that managers, simply because they are managers, must adopt certain patterns of behavior when doing management work.

He saw the work of managers as a series of three broad categories of roles—interpersonal, informational, and decisional—with each category composed of a number of separate and distinct roles as summarized in Figure 1.5.

FIGURE 1.5. THE MANAGER'S ROLES.

- **Interpersonal Roles**
  - Figurehead
  - Influencer (leader)
  - Liaison
- **Informational Roles**
  - Monitor
  - Disseminator
  - Spokesperson
- **Decisional Roles**
  - Entreprenuer
  - Disturbance handler
  - Resource allocator
  - Negotiator

Interpersonal Roles. In Mintzberg's view, all managers play *interpersonal roles* as figurehead, influencer or leader, and liaison. The figurehead role is played as managers engage in ceremonial and symbolic activities such as presiding over the opening of an additional site for a program or giving a speech to a graduating class of speech pathology students. Managers play their influencer or leader roles when they seek to inspire or help others to be motivated to higher levels of performance or when they set examples through their own behavior. Liaison roles involve managers making formal and informal contacts inside their program or project and also with external stakeholders. Managers usually pursue liaison roles in order to establish relationships that will help them achieve the program or project's mission and objectives.

Informational Roles. As Figure 1.5 illustrates, Mintzberg also ascribes a category of *informational roles* to managers in which they serve as monitors, disseminators, and spokespersons. In their monitor roles, managers gather information from their networks of contacts—including those established in their liaison roles—filter the information, evaluate it, and choose how to act as a result of the information. Their disseminator roles grow out of access to information and their ability to choose what to do with the information they obtain. In dissemination, managers have many choices about whom, inside and outside their programs or projects, they route information to. The third informational role, the spokesperson role, is related to managers' figurehead roles. As spokespeople, managers communicate information about their programs or projects to internal and external stakeholders.

Decisional Roles. The third category of roles managers play in Mintzberg's model, *decisional roles,* includes entrepreneur, disturbance handler, resource allocator, and negotiator roles. In their roles as entrepreneurs, managers function as initiators and designers of changes intended to improve performance in their programs or projects. When playing this role, managers are acting as change agents. In their disturbance handler roles, managers decide how to handle a wide variety of disturbances (for example problems or issues) that arise as they carry out their daily work routines. A program manager may face disturbances created by participants, by a regulatory agency, or by the actions of a competitor. Even a heavy snowfall that makes it impossible for key participants to come to work can be a significant disturbance. The ability to handle disturbances is an important determinant of managerial success in programs and projects.

In playing the resource allocator role, managers must allocate human and other resources among alternative uses. As resources become constrained, decisions about resource allocation become more difficult and more important. In their negotiator roles, managers interact and bargain with participants, suppliers, regulators, customers or patients, and others who have some relationship to their program or project. Negotiating includes deciding what objectives or outcomes to seek through negotiation, as well as deciding what techniques will be used in conducting the negotiations they enter.

The ten managerial roles shown in Figure 1.5 cannot really be neatly separated. In practice, they are closely intertwined into a *gestalt,* or an integrated whole. Management work is not merely the algebraic sum of these ten roles, but is much more. When the interconnected roles are each played well, the result is synergistic. Being a good negotiator makes a manager a better disturbance handler. Playing the informational roles effectively improves performance in the decisional roles because this provides managers with better information upon which to base their decisions.

Most, if not all, of the activities managers engage in as they manage their programs and projects can be categorized into one or more of the core or facilitative activities depicted in Figure 1.4. Similarly, the roles managers play are comprehensively summarized in Figure 1.5. However, descriptions of these activities and roles say very little about the *skills* or *competencies* needed to perform the activities or play the roles well. Thus, another important element in understanding management work is to understand the skills and competencies upon which successful managers rely.

Skills and Competencies That Underpin Management Work

Katz (1974) has identified three types of skills effective managers use: technical, conceptual, and human or interpersonal. The *technical skills* of managers, like the technical skills of a physical therapist or a nurse, are apparent as they do their work. A manager's work to counsel a participant in a program about performance, or develop a budget for a project requires technical skills. *Human or interpersonal skills* are the abilities of managers to get along with other people, to understand them, and to lead them in the workplace. *Conceptual skills* reflect the mental abilities of managers to visualize the complex interrelationships that exist in a workplace. For example, relationships may exist between and among a program and other departments or units in its organizational home. Relationships may also exist between participants in a program and other components of the external environment. Conceptual skills permit managers to understand how factors in particular situations fit together and interact with one another. Conceptual skills are clearly reflected in the quality of a program or project's logic model and organization design.

Managers Use Different Mixes of Skills. Not all managers use conceptual, technical, and human skills to the same degree or in the same mix, although every manager relies on all three types of skills in performing management work. For example, the management work that takes place in a very large program providing health education services could require three different levels of management and three different mixes of technical, human, and conceptual skills. The program manager would be vitally concerned about the overall performance of the program and how it fits within its larger environment. If this program were housed in a hospital, for example, the manager would be concerned about how the program fits into the total picture of the hospital and its plans, including how the program might grow in the future. Such concerns would require a heavy dependence on conceptual skills.

The large health education program might have major subdivisions (such as one that focuses on services offered to individual clients and another to provide services to employers for their employees), each with its own division director. These middle-level managers would rely more on their technical skills than on conceptual or human skills, although like all managers they would use all the skills to a degree. In this program the division managers spend much of their time troubleshooting the health education services provided by their division; they may be required to constantly make decisions on the basis of technical knowledge.

In contrast to the program manager and the two division directors, a health educator who is the account manager in charge of a team providing services to a single employer might use a considerable amount of technical skill because in addition to being a first-level manager, this individual must provide health education services. However, this manager would also be required to use human skills on the job more than either the program manager or the division directors, because almost all of this person's work involves direct contact with the other educators on the team. This variation in the mixes of these three types of skills used in management work can be seen in Figure 1.6.

Competencies Needed to Manage Effectively

Longest (1998a) extends the Katz model of skills required of managers to a broader set of what are called *competencies,* which he defines as clusters of knowledge and skill in using the knowledge. In this somewhat broader approach, with

FIGURE 1.6. RELATIVE MIXES OF SKILLS NEEDED FOR EFFECTIVE
MANAGEMENT WORK IN A LARGE PROGRAM.

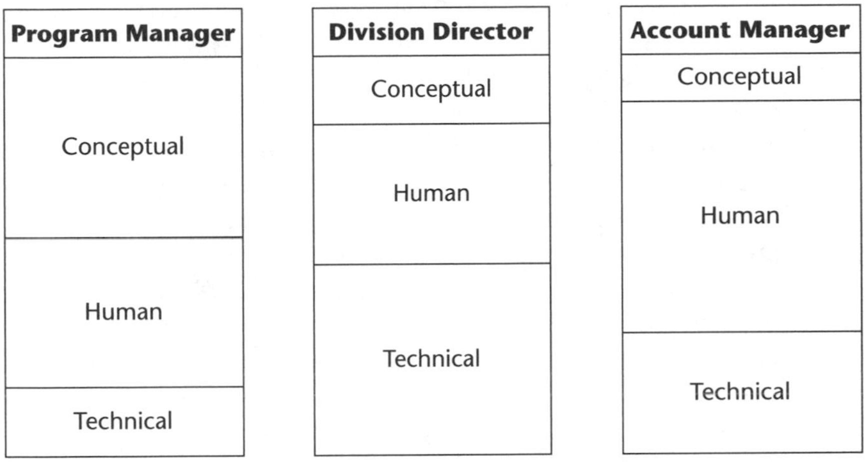

Program Manager	Division Director	Account Manager
Conceptual	Conceptual	Conceptual
	Human	Human
Human		
	Technical	
Technical		Technical

some overlap with the Katz model, the competencies useful to program and project managers are as follows:

- Conceptual
- Technical (managerial and clinical)
- Interpersonal and collaborative
- Political
- Commercial

Governance is also a useful competency for those whose programs or projects are freestanding rather than embedded in larger organizations.

Conceptual Competency. In all settings, managers must be able to envision the places and roles of their programs or projects within their larger contexts. This may mean envisioning places and roles in the larger society, as well as in the organizational home in which a program or project is embedded. This competency also allows managers to visualize the complex interrelationships in their workplaces—relationships among participants within a program or project, as well as relationships of the program or project to other units of an organization or external entities with which it interacts. In short, adequate conceptual competency allows managers to identify, understand, and interact with their program or project's myriad external and internal stakeholders. *Conceptual* competency also enhances a manager's ability to comprehend the culture and historically developed values, beliefs, and norms present in the program or project, and to visualize its future.

Technical (Managerial and Clinical) Competency. The cluster of knowledge and associated skills that make up *technical* competency pertains to management work as well as to the direct work performed in a program or project. In health programs and projects, direct work often involves clinical activities such as conducting a health education session, performing a screening test, conducting a physical therapy session, or counseling a patient. The technical aspects of management work, such as planning for a new service or facility or developing a program or project budget, are also crucial to the program or project's success. Knowledge and relevant skills in using or applying the knowledge in both clinical and management areas make up technical competency for health program and project managers.

Interpersonal and Collaborative Competency. An important ingredient in managerial success is the cluster of knowledge and related skills about human interactions and relations by which managers lead others in pursuit of a program or project's mission and objectives. A survey of managers to determine competencies most important to success in management performance in ambulatory health services settings found interpersonal skills rated most highly (Hudak, Brooke, Finstuen, and Trounson 1997). *Interpersonal* competency incorporates knowledge and skills useful in effectively interacting with others. It enables managers to help participants achieve higher levels of motivation and handle conflicts among participants.

The core elements of traditional interpersonal competence expand considerably when programs or projects must interact with other organizational entities. This requires *collaborative* competency, which facilitates synergistic interaction among programs, projects, and various other organizational units. Collaborative competency is exercised when, for example, two programs are successfully merged, or when a joint venture among programs is created and operated to better serve a particular population. This competency relies upon a manager's ability to build trust among programs, projects, and other organizational units, and to effectively form partnerships with other units to achieve certain purposes. It also is reflected in the ability to build effective coalitions and alliances.

Political Competency. *Political* competency, defined as the dual capability to accurately assess the impact of public policies on the performance of a program or project *and* to influence public policy making at state and federal levels (Longest 1996; 2002), is an increasingly important competency for program and project managers. Managers can influence public policy at many points in the policy-making process. For example, they can help define problems that policies can address; they can help create solutions to the problems; or they can help establish the political circumstances necessary to advance solutions through the policy-making process (Kingdon 1995).

Program and project managers are often in excellent positions to know first-hand about particular health problems because they deal with them daily. Similarly, by permitting their program or project to serve as a demonstration site (for assessing possible solutions), they can play important roles in identifying feasible solutions to problems.

Based on their knowledge and expertise in addressing particular health issues, managers can participate in drafting legislative proposals and testify at legislative hearings. They can also influence rule making. Procedurally, rule making typically precedes and guides the implementation of public policies and is designed to include input in the form of formal comments on proposed rules from those who will be affected by them.

Commercial Competency. In any setting, *commercial* competency is the ability of managers to establish and operate value-creating situations in which economic exchanges between buyers and sellers occur. Value in health services has a specific meaning. It requires that buyers and sellers think about both *quality* and *price.* Value is quality divided by price. Value in the services produced by most health programs or projects is created when services have more of the quality attributes desired by buyers than competitors offer. Value is also created when a program or project can produce and sell a set of quality attributes at a lower price than its competitors. The commercial success of health programs and projects may be essential for their survival. This success requires managers to possess commercial competency.

Governance Competency. When programs and projects are embedded in larger organizations, the organization's governing board is relevant to the program or project in the same way it is relevant to other units in the organization. Managers of such programs or projects may have little need for *governance* competency. However, when health programs and projects exist as freestanding entities they may have their own governing boards. In these situations, governance competency is also important for their managers.

The governing board, in concert with the manager, is responsible for establishing a clear vision for the program or project, for fostering a culture that supports the realization of the vision, for assembling and effectively allocating the resources to realize the vision, for leading the program, project, or organization through various challenges in its external environment, and for ensuring proper accountability to multiple stakeholders (Orlikoff and Totten 1996).

When programs and projects have governing boards of their own, the knowledge and associated skills that make up governance competency are important for their managers for three reasons. First, in freestanding programs and projects, managers often participate directly in the governance function as members of its governing body. Second, at the top level of a program or project it is difficult to separate what occurs under the rubric of governance from what occurs as management work. Consequently, effective managers must be knowledgeable about management *and* governance. Third, managers can help those with direct governance responsibilities to do a better job by arranging educational activities for board members or by providing appropriate information to help with governance.

The work of managers has been viewed from the perspective of the activities managers engage in as they do their work (see Figure 1.4), and from the perspective of the managerial roles they play in doing management work (see Figure 1.5). Each perspective contributes to an understanding of management work. In addition, it is also important to consider the ethical aspects of management work.

Managing Programs and Projects Ethically

The beginning of an appreciation for the extent to which ethics affects management work rests in the recognition that all decisions and actions in health programs and projects include ethics dimensions, whether they are clinical or managerial decisions, or some combination. Managers, if they are to behave ethically, must first recognize ethical issues and then act on them.

Managers routinely make decisions and take actions that have consequences for their programs or projects, as well as for their internal and external stakeholders. As a foundation for their decisions and actions, managers need well-developed personal ethics standards, which must be applied in the context of the philosophy and culture of the program or project, and in many instances in the context of the philosophy and culture of the organization in which it is embedded. Compatibility between the personal ethics standards of managers and those of the programs, projects, and organizations within which they work is important, and both sets of standards should be built upon four key ethics principles: respect for persons, justice, beneficence, and nonmaleficence.

Respect for Persons

The principle of *respect for persons* has four elements: autonomy of persons, truth telling, confidentiality, and fidelity. The concept of autonomy recognizes that individuals have the right to their own beliefs and values and to the decisions and choices that further these beliefs and values. Specifically, autonomy pertains to the rights of individuals to independent self-determination regarding how they live their lives; autonomy also pertains to the rights of individuals regarding what happens to them in health care situations.

In health programs or projects, honoring the autonomy of patients/customers means following their wishes about their care and letting them be involved in their care to the extent they choose to be. It also means that when its patients/customers are children or are adults of diminished competence through physical or mental condition, the program or project has special procedures for surrogate decision making or substituted judgments.

The principle of respect for persons is especially important in its effect on consent and use of confidential patient information in health programs and projects. Respect for persons as autonomous beings implies honesty in relationships with them. Closely related to honesty in such relationships is the element of confidentiality. Confidences broken will impair the performance of management work.

A fourth element of the respect for persons is fidelity. This means doing one's duty and keeping one's word. Fidelity is often equated with promise keeping. When managers tell the truth, honor confidences, and keep promises, they are behaving in an ethically sound manner.

Decisions and actions that reflect the principle of respect for persons can sometimes be better understood in contrast to its opposite—paternalism. Paternalism implies that someone else knows what is best for other people. Decisions and actions guided by a preference for autonomy limit paternalism. One of the most vivid examples of the application of this principle in health care is the 1990 Patient Self-Determination Act (Public Law 101-508). This public policy is designed to give individuals the right to make decisions concerning their health care, including the right to accept or refuse treatment and the right to formulate advance directives regarding their care. These directives are a means by which competent individuals give instructions about their health care that are to be implemented at some later date should they lack the capacity to make these decisions. In concept, this policy gave people the right to exercise their autonomy in advance of a time when they might no longer be able to actively exercise the right.

Justice

A second ethics principle of significant importance to managers and their work in programs and projects is *justice.* The concept of justice impacts directly on management work because justice, in the context of ethics, is defined as fairness (Rawls 1999). The principle of justice also includes the concept of desert: justice is done when a person receives that which he or she deserves (Beauchamp and Childress 2001). The key ethical question in many of the decisions and actions of managers, deriving from attention to the principle of justice, is, of course, "What is fair in this situation?"

The principle of justice provides much of the underpinning for ethically sound decisions and actions regarding the allocation of resources. Decisions about resource allocation that adhere closely to the principle of justice are made under the provisions of a morally defensible system and are not arbitrary or capricious. The application of justice in activities of making decisions in health programs and projects, as well as in other settings, is in part ensured by the existence of the legal system. This system serves as an appeals mechanism for those who believe they have been done an injustice.

Beneficence and Nonmaleficence

Two other ethics principles have direct relevance to managers in health programs and projects: beneficence and nonmaleficence. *Beneficence* means acting with charity and kindness. This principle is incorporated into acts through which services or products are provided that are beneficial to people, including the services of health programs and projects. However, the principle of beneficence also includes the more complex concept of balancing benefits and harms, which may require using the relative costs and benefits of alternative decisions and actions as one basis upon which to choose from among alternatives.

The growing emphasis on cost-effectiveness in health care will increasingly call into play the principle of beneficence in the conduct of management work in health programs and projects. Managers who are guided by the principle of beneficence feel a positive duty to contribute to the welfare of patients/customers. This is rooted in the Hippocratic tradition and has a long and noble history in the health professions and in health care settings, including health programs and projects.

Nonmaleficence, a principle with deep roots in medical ethics, is exemplified in the dictum *primum non nocere,* which means, first, do no harm. Managers who are guided by the principle of nonmaleficence try to make decisions that minimize harm. Harm can be mental as well as physical and can be caused through such acts as violating the privacy of patients/customers. While beneficence is a positive duty involving taking action to do good, nonmaleficence involves refraining from doing something that harms. The principles of beneficence and nonmaleficence are reflected in actions and decisions to assure the quality of the services of a program or project. These principles are also reflected in managers' exercise of their fiduciary duties, use of confidential information, and resolution of conflicts of interest.

Supporting Ethical Behavior in Health Programs and Projects

Health programs and projects, by their nature, frequently involve health professionals providing health services. In these situations, the professionals face a set of ethical obligations that stem from their roles as professionals. These obligations have been described by Bayles (1989) and are summarized in the following categories:

Obligations to make services available	This obligation requires equality of opportunity in access to professional services. Ethical issues arise in the form of access problems such as what to do about patients/customers who cannot pay for services.
Obligations between professionals and patients/customers	"The fiduciary model presents the best ethical ideal for the professional-client relationship" (Bayles 1989, p. 100). In this model, the professional is honest, candid, competent, loyal, fair, and discreet in relationships with patients/customers.

Obligations to third parties

In many health programs and projects, other people or organizations (for example parents or other family members, employers, teachers, insurance plans) have interests in the professional-patient or professional-customer relationship. The ethical issues that arise from these obligations usually involve issues of confidentiality and the protection of privacy. These issues often involve complying with laws such as the Health Insurance Portability and Accountability Act (HIPAA). They may also involve responding to court orders. HIPAA, enacted by Congress in 1997, includes privacy provisions that generally limit the use or disclosure of protected health information to a minimum necessary standard (Harris 2003, pp. 108–120). It also gives patients the right to see and receive copies of their records, request amendments to their records, and learn details about disclosures of their records.

Obligations between professionals and their employers

Obligations exist between professionals and the health programs and projects that employ them. In some cases, these obligations also exist between professionals and the larger organizational homes in which programs or projects are embedded. Ethical issues that arise from these obligations involve due process, confidentiality, and professional support. Professionals, as participants, have obligations to their employers that include being honest, candid, competent, loyal, fair, and discreet.

Obligations to the profession   The professionals who work in health programs and projects have obligations to their professions that include advancing knowledge, reforming the profession, and respecting the profession. These obligations "rest on the responsibilities of a profession as a whole to further social values" (Bayles 1989, p. 179).

A number of codes of ethics have been developed for individual professions, as well as for various health care organizations. For example, the American Hospital Association has produced a prototype code of ethics for hospitals. It includes sections on the community roles and responsibilities of these institutions, on patient care in them, and on organizational conduct. The American Medical Association adopted the first version of its *Principles of Medical Ethics* at its founding in 1847. The American Nurses Association has developed a code for nurses. The American College of Healthcare Executives has produced a code of ethics to guide members on ethical issues. Similarly, other health professions have developed codes. In fact, a code of ethics is a hallmark of any profession. Beyond these codes, many individual health care organizations develop their own codes. These often provide very visible evidence of the commitment of organizations to ethical behavior; programs and projects embedded in such organizations can also use these codes of ethics.

In addition to relying upon codes of ethical behavior developed by others, a program or project-specific code of ethical behavior can provide specific guidelines for participants to follow. Managers can support ethical behavior in other ways as well. They can develop cultures within their programs or projects that minimize ethical ambiguity and continuously remind participants to make ethical decisions and take ethical actions. They can reward ethical behavior and create climates in which people are free to challenge standards or practices they consider unethical. Finally, they can encourage ethical behavior by providing training in applied ethics in order to increase awareness of the ethical dimensions of decisions and actions, encourage critical evaluations of values and priorities, and help participants integrate ethical considerations into their decisions and actions.

Managers and the Success of Programs and Projects

To conclude this introductory chapter, it is important to emphasize the significant impact that managers can have on their programs and projects. Health programs and projects are not random groups of people assembled by chance interactions. Instead, they are consciously formed around a logic model. From this fact stems the overarching purpose of all management work in a program or project, which is to facilitate the achievement of its intended results, whether expressed as outputs, outcomes, or impact.

The contributions managers make to the degree to which desired results are successfully accomplished can be measured along many dimensions. Measuring their overall contributions to success may involve measuring a program or project's *outputs* in terms of counts of services and productivity levels, quality of services, and patient/customer satisfaction. For example, the number of services rendered can be counted and compared to established targets. Productivity can be measured in terms of resources used per unit of service. Quality of the services provided by a program or project can be measured in terms of clinical outcomes achieved, as well as process measures such as adherence to protocols and input measures such as the credentials of staff. Patient/customer satisfaction levels can be measured by surveys and by loyalty demonstrated by continued use of services.

In addition to outputs, a manager's contributions to a program or project's success can also be measured in terms of *outcomes,* such as changes in the attitudes, behaviors, health status, or level of functioning in patients/customers. Finally, managers' contributions can be measured in terms of *impact* of the program or project on overall health status in a community, for example, or on the enhanced capacity of a health care organization in which a program or project is housed to respond to unmet service needs in a community.

There is no universally accepted formula by which managers maximize their contributions to program and project effectiveness. However, there is a correlation between a program or project's success and how well its manager performs the core activities of designing, strategizing, and leading. Similarly, the manner in which a manager makes decisions, communicates, manages change and quality, and markets the program or project may have a direct bearing on success.

There is also a correlation between the use of appropriate mixes of conceptual, human or interpersonal, and technical skills by managers and the degree to which desired results are attained. Similarly, performance is affected by a program or project manager's possession and use of appropriate conceptual, technical (managerial and clinical), interpersonal and collaborative, political, commercial, and governance competencies. Finally, there is a correlation between how well managers play their interpersonal, informational, and decisional roles and the levels of performance their programs and projects attain. Effective managers, by creating conditions that are conducive to superior performance, make vital and unique contributions to the programs and projects they manage. The remaining chapters in this book are intended to help managers maximize their contributions to successful programs and projects.

Summary

Definitions of health, health programs and projects, and management are provided in this chapter. Following the World Health Organization's view—and more contemporary interpretations of it—health is defined as a state in which the biological and clinical indicators of organ function are maximized and in which physical, mental, and role functioning in everyday life are also maximized.

Health is a function of a number of health determinants, which for individuals or populations include the following:

- The physical environments in which people live and work
- Peoples' behaviors
- Peoples' biology (genetic makeup and physical and mental health problems acquired during life)
- A host of social factors that include economic circumstances, socioeconomic position in society, and income distribution
- Discrimination based on factors such as race or ethnicity, gender, or sexual orientation
- The availability of social networks and social support
- The health services to which people have access

The variety of health determinants means that health programs and projects can have a wide array of foci.

Health programs are defined as discrete sets of interrelated people and other resources arranged in designs that facilitate accomplishment of pre-established results. Health projects are a subset of programs that tend to be more time-limited than other programs and are often supported by project-specific grants. The usefulness of considering a program and project in terms of its logic model, which shows how inputs and resources are processed to accomplish the program or project's outputs, outcomes, and ultimately its impact, is emphasized. Viewing programs and projects as organizations is also discussed.

Program or project management is defined as the activities through which the desired outputs, outcomes, and impact of a program or project are established and pursued through various processes using human and other resources. Following the basic logic model of a program or project (see Figure 1.1), managers, often with the help of others accomplish the following:

- Determine a program or project's desired outputs, outcomes, and impact
- Assemble the necessary inputs and resources to achieve desired results
- Determine the processes necessary to accomplish the desired results and ensure they are carried out effectively and efficiently
- Relate the program or project to its external environment

The work of managers is considered in terms of the core activities that all managers engage in as they do management work: strategizing, designing, and leading. Consideration of this work is extended to include the facilitative activities managers engage in as they perform management work, including decision making, communicating, managing quality, and marketing. The entire set of core and facilitative activities in management work is presented graphically in Figure 1.4. The core and facilitative activities of management work form the chapter outline for the remainder of this book.

As an adjunct to the discussion of the activities in management work, Mintzberg's model of the roles that managers play in doing management work is also presented. Figure 1.5 summarizes these roles in interpersonal, informational, and decisional categories. There is also a discussion of the conceptual, technical, and human skills that are useful to managers in doing their work, as well as the conceptual, technical (managerial and clinical), interpersonal and collaborative, political, commercial, and governance competencies that can be useful in performing management work.

The chapter acknowledges the growing impact that ethical considerations have on all actions and decisions in health programs and projects in both the clinical and management spheres of activity. The ethical principles of respect for persons, justice, beneficence, and nonmaleficence are discussed as the basis for the construction of a personal and professional ethic for managers.

The chapter concludes by noting the correlation between a program or project's success and how well its manager performs the core and facilitative activities of designing, strategizing, leading, decision making, and communicating. A program or project's success is also affected by how well its manager manages quality and markets the program or project.

Chapter Review Questions

1. Define health, health programs and projects, and management.
2. Discuss how the determinants of health shape the focus of health programs and projects.
3. Briefly describe the core activities of management work.
4. Briefly describe the facilitative activities of management work.
5. Discuss the skills that are useful to managers in performing their work, including the different mixes of skills that would be appropriate in different circumstances.
6. Discuss the competencies managers need if they are to do their work well.
7. Discuss the Mintzberg model of the roles managers play in doing their work.
8. Why is it important for managers to develop personal ethical standards of conduct? Discuss the principles upon which such standards should be based.
9. Discuss the overall contributions managers make to the success of the health programs and projects they manage.

EXAMPLE OF A HEALTH PROGRAM

Connecting Lifestyle and Health: A Grassroots Program Reaches Out to a Specific Community Group

Scott Reiner, President and Chief Executive Officer, Glendale Adventist Medical Center

At Glendale (CA) Adventist Medical Center, our mission statement promotes "healing, health, and wellness for the whole person." We know that patients who come through our doors every day can benefit tremendously from this approach to healthcare. But it doesn't end there. What about the people in our community who have not yet accessed our hospital's services? We believe that we have a commitment to them as well. That's why our mission statement also includes the phrase "working together with our community." Glendale Adventist's Hearts N' Health program is an excellent example of this commitment. Through an approach that expands the boundaries of traditional healthcare, Hearts N' Health teaches local Armenian-American residents about the connection between their lifestyle behaviors and their health.

A Simple Beginning

The impetus for Hearts N' Health was an ordinary circumstance—a health fair. In 1992, Glendale Adventist and the Armenian American Medical Society sponsored a health fair for local Armenian-Americans, who make up approximately 30 percent of Glendale's community. At this health fair and other screenings, we discovered that the majority of participants were new immigrants whose lifestyles put them at higher risk for health problems such as obesity and heart disease. Some of the more prevalent behavior issues included:

- High levels of stress—Stress is exacerbated by the intergenerational conflict faced by immigrants raising their children in American culture.
- Lack of exercise—Regular exercise is generally not part of the Armenian lifestyle.
- Poor food choices—The typical Armenian diet is high in fat and calories.

Most troubling of all was that health fair participants didn't see the connection between what they did and how healthy they were. To compound the problem, a majority had never even accessed the health care system. As a result, Glendale Adventist's leaders decided that we needed to offer better health intervention services to the Armenian-American community.

A Unique Approach

Glendale Adventist teamed up with a number of local Armenian-American organizations: the Armenian American Medical Society, Armenian Nursing Association, Armenian Relief Society, Glendale City Armenian Church, Armenian Advisory Council for Glendale Adventist, and Southern California Adventist Health Network. After discussing different strategies for a year, we started Hearts N' Health, a program that focuses on educating Armenian-Americans about cardiac fitness, stress management, smoking cessation, exercise, and proper nutrition.

With the help of our Armenian-American community partners, we identified twelve local Armenian women who wanted to teach their peers about key health issues. These volunteer health educators were then trained by a team made up of a program coordinator (manager), physical therapist, public health educator, and registered dietitian, who used instruction manuals with pictures and other visual aids. Armed with this training and specially developed materials written in Armenian, each lay educator goes into the homes of local Armenian-Americans. A hostess invites friends and family to hear the educator's presentation. At the end, participants are asked if any of them would like to be a hostess, and the process is repeated with the new hostess and different guests. This grassroots method reaches more than 500 people each year!

The lay educator approach is particularly suited to Armenian culture not only because people can learn better in their own language, but also because informal communication works well in a community that has tight-knit extended families. In addition, the Hearts N' Health presentations enable educators to easily reach other Armenian women, who typically make most of the decisions about healthy habits and food choices for their families.

To expand its educational efforts, Hearts N' Health launched the Armenian-language television show *Healthy Families* in 2001. Hosted by Hovik Sarrafian, Ph.D., a respected Armenian public health educator, this program airs on public access cable TV and reaches 10,000 viewers every week. Each one-hour program features two segments: a discussion of a specific health topic and a call-in portion that allows viewers to ask questions.

To date, 135 shows have aired, featuring topics such as weight management, depression, back pain, and nutrition. And the program's call-in line now receives more than seventy calls per show. Since the cable channel is largely devoted to Armenian programming, community members already identify with it, making them more likely to watch *Healthy Families*.

Because Hearts N' Health implements an approach that is tailored to their culture, Armenian-American residents have become more open to making lifestyle changes that improve their health, such as managing stress, exercising, eating less fat, reading food labels, and getting regular physicals. In fact, more than 90 percent of respondents in a 2002 random survey indicated that the in-home presentations and other program features have positively affected their lifestyle.

The Next Step

Glendale Adventist plans to use the Hearts N' Health model to reach other minority populations. Our goal continues to be partnering with individuals in an ethnic group to address their unique situation, instead of simply going to them and saying, "This is what we're going to do for you." As the Hearts N' Health program had demonstrated, we can improve community health—working together.

Source: Used with permission from *Healthcare Executive,* the official magazine of the American College of Healthcare Executives. (Vol. 18, No. 6): 52–53.

EXAMPLE OF A HEALTH PROJECT

National Standards for Culturally and Linguistically Appropriate Services in Health Care

Office of Minority Health, U.S. Department of Health and Human Services

As the U.S. Population becomes more diverse, medical providers and other people involved in health care delivery are interacting with patients or consumers from many different cultural and linguistic backgrounds. Because culture and language are vital factors in how health care services are delivered and received, it is important that health care organizations and their staff understand and respond with sensitivity to the needs and preferences that culturally and linguistically diverse patients or consumers bring to the health encounter. Providing culturally and linguistically appropriate services (CLAS) to these patients has the potential to improve access to care, quality of care, and, ultimately, health outcomes.

Unfortunately, a lack of comprehensive standards has left organizations and providers with no clear guidance on how to provide CLAS in health care settings. In 1997, the Office of Minority Health (OMH) undertook the development of national standards to provide a much-needed alternative to the current patchwork of independently developed definitions, practices, and requirements concerning CLAS. The Office initiated a project to develop recommended national CLAS standards that would support a more consistent and comprehensive approach to cultural and linguistic competence in health care.

The first stage of the project involved a review and analysis of existing cultural and linguistic competence standards and measures, the development of draft standards, and revisions based on a review by a national advisory committee. The second stage focused on obtaining and incorporating input from organizations, agencies, and individuals that have a vital stake in the establishment of CLAS standards. Publication of standards in the *Federal Register* on December 15, 1999, announced a four-month public comment period, which provided three regional meetings and a Web site as well as traditional avenues (mail and fax) for submitting feedback on the CLAS standards. A project team (consisting of staff members of OMH, its contractor, and subcontractor) analyzed public comments from 413 individuals or organizations and proposed revised standards, with accompanying commentaries, to a National Project Advisory Committee (NPAC). Deliberations and additional review by NPAC members informed further refinements of the standards.

In their final version, the CLAS standards reflect input from a broad range of stakeholders, including hospitals, community-based clinics, managed care organizations, home health agencies, and other types of health care organizations; physicians, nurses, and other providers; professional associations; state and federal agencies and other policymakers; purchasers of health care; accreditation and credentialing agencies; educators; and patient advocates, advocacy groups, and consumers.

The CLAS standards were published in final form in the *Federal Register* on December 22, 2000, as recommended national standards for adoption or adaptation by stakeholder organizations and agencies.

Source: Office of Minority Health, U.S. Department of Health and Human Services. "Project Overview," *National Standards for Culturally and Linguistically Appropriate Services in Health Care*. Washington, D. C.: Office of Minority Health, U.S. Department of Health and Human Services (March 2001): 1.

CHAPTER TWO

STRATEGIZING THE FUTURE

Managers engage in three highly interrelated core activities as they perform management work: *strategizing, designing,* and *leading* (see Figure 1.3). When managers, often with the involvement of others, establish the desired results to be achieved through a program or project and conceptualize the means of accomplishing the results, they are *strategizing*. Through strategizing, managers establish the desired outputs, outcomes, and impact for a program or project (as shown in Figure 1.1) and develop appropriate operational plans to accomplish them.

Through *strategizing* activities, managers lay a foundation for *designing* the inputs and processes or components of a program or project's logic model (see Figure 1.1). Strategizing activities also help managers design intentional patterns of relationships among the human and other resources within the program or project. The desired results established through strategizing the future of a program or project, along with the operational plans as to how to accomplish the desired results, also inform managers about where they should be *leading* other participants.

Strategizing for a nascent program or project requires managers to engage in different activities than when strategizing for an ongoing project or program. Both situations are covered in this chapter, although the more common situation of strategizing in ongoing programs and projects receives more attention. The special circumstance of the initial round of strategizing for a new program or project being developed is discussed in terms of preparing a *business plan* for it, which includes developing the original logic model for the program or project as well as other aspects about how it will operate.

In an ongoing program or project, managers strategize, often with the involvement of other participants, in order to answer four critical questions about their programs or projects:

1. What is the current situation of our program or project?
2. In what ways do we want our program or project's situation to change in the future?
3. How will we move our program or project to the preferred future state?
4. Are we making acceptable progress toward the desired future state?

This chapter provides information about how managers can answer these four key questions. The chapter discusses how question number one is answered through the conduct of what we will call an *internal* and *external situational analysis* for a program or project, as well as the development of an inventory of the desired results established for it. The chapter discusses how question number two is answered through reconsideration of the components of a program or project's logic model, which include inputs and resources, processes, outputs, outcomes, and impact. We will discuss how revisions in logic models and organization designs serve as the mechanism to answer question number three. Revisions may involve changing any part of a program or project's inputs, processes, and desired results, and may require detailed *operational planning*. Techniques of assessing and controlling performance and evaluating results are discussed as the mechanisms to answer question number four about programs and projects. After reading the chapter, the reader should be able to do the following:

- Understand how to conduct internal and external situational analyses
- Formulate and reformulate statements of desired outputs, outcomes, and impact for a program or project
- Model the operational planning process and understand the steps in the process
- Understand how to assess and control performance and evaluate results to achieve the desired results established for a program or project

Health programs and projects typically operate within the context of extremely turbulent external environments; managers must therefore be prepared to accept uncertainty as the inevitable consequence of operating in such a dynamic world. However, managers have a responsibility to try to reduce the uncertainty and prepare their programs or projects to cope with it. As managers seek to reduce and otherwise cope with uncertainty, effective strategizing is often their most useful and powerful tool. They engage in strategizing activities in order to answer the four questions presented earlier in this section.

What Is the Current Situation of Our Program or Project?

Conducting a Situational Analysis

Effective strategizing in an ongoing program or project should be based on the periodic conduct of a thorough *situational analysis,* in which available information about the current situation of a program or project is collected and analyzed. The eventual effectiveness of strategizing activities depends upon the quality and quantity of the information generated through situational analysis. In practice, situational analysis is ongoing, although it is useful to complete the entire analysis at least once during each year of operation.

A thorough situational analysis for a program or project includes three components: an *external situational analysis,* an *internal situational analysis,* and *an inventory of the desired results* established for the program or project. The inventory can be organized into desired outputs, outcomes, and impact as shown in logic models (see Figure 1.1).

A manager's complete situational analysis considers the results intended for a program or project in relation to opportunities and threats in the external environment and also in relation to the internal strengths and weaknesses of the program or project. Sometimes the internal and external situational analyses are termed a *SWOT analysis,* an acronym derived from the fact that the analysis is conducted to determine a program or project's **s**trengths, **w**eaknesses, **o**pportunities, and **t**hreats. SWOT is among the most widely used analytical tools in strategizing, because it is intuitive and relatively simple to use (Luke, Walston, and Plummer 2004).

The order in which the external and internal analyses are made in the situational analysis is important because most internal strengths and weaknesses can be identified only in relation to the external environment. For example, a health program's physical location can be considered one of its strengths if its services are in demand in the area in which it is located. Otherwise, physical location may be a weakness for a program or project. Answering the question, "What is the current situation of our program or project?" begins with the external situational analysis.

External Situational Analysis

A program or project's external environment produces combinations of demographic, economic, legal, policy, social, and technological information that, depending upon circumstances, may be relevant to its future. All health programs and projects can be influenced, sometimes dramatically, by what goes on in their external environments. External environments can provide health programs and projects with both opportunities and threats. Both opportunities and threats must be identified for effective strategizing to take place.

The relevant external environment includes all the factors outside a program or project's boundaries that can influence its manager's decisions and actions. Factors may include complementary or competitive programs and projects; an organizational home if the program or project is embedded in an organization; as well as patients/customers, suppliers, regulators, insurers, accrediting agencies and so on with which the program or project has direct interactions. The relevant external environment also includes other more general aspects of the external environment that can have a direct or indirect impact on the program or project. Thus the general economy, the policy-making system, the legal system, the physical environment, and cultural norms and patterns are relevant.

The conduct of an external situational analysis includes five interrelated steps: (1) scanning to identify relevant information (trends, developments, or possible events that represent either opportunities or threats for the program or project); (2) monitoring or tracking the relevant information identified through scanning; (3) forecasting or projecting the future directions of relevant information; (4) assessing the implications of the information for the program or project; and (5) disseminating the information to those who can use it to guide decisions and actions (Ginter, Swayne, and Duncan 2002). Each of these steps is discussed next.

Scanning. Scanning the external environment of a program or project involves acquiring and organizing information that can affect its future. The effect might be felt in any part of the program or project's logic model (see Figure 1.1). That is, the effect could be on inputs available to the program or project or to its conduct of processes to achieve desired results. Information can even change its desired results. An outcome objective of reducing teenage pregnancies, for example, could be affected when demographic shifts in a program or project's community result in fewer teenagers.

Determining what is important to scan is often a matter of judgment. For this reason, it is useful to have more than one person making these judgments. One widely used approach to decide what information is relevant is to involve other people in the judgments. For example, a manager might rely upon a group of participants in a program or project to decide what to scan. If there is a larger organizational home, the group may include some members from it. Another useful approach is to use outside consultants to provide expert opinions and judgments.

Although the determination of what is important to scan is specific to a particular program or project, there are models designed to guide the conduct of situational analyses. One model that is especially useful in conducting a situational analysis or assessment at the level of an entire community is the Mobilizing for Action Through Planning and Partnerships (MAPP) model. This model, which has been developed by the National Association of County and City Health Officials (NACCHO) in cooperation with the Public Health Practice Program Office of the Centers for Disease Control and Prevention (CDC), can be reviewed at http://mapp.naccho.org. As noted on this Web site, the MAPP model (http://mapp.naccho.org/fulltextintroduction.asp) relies on the following four different assessments to gather situational information at the level of a community:

The Community Themes and Strengths Assessment	Identifies themes that interest and engage the community, perceptions about quality of life, and community assets
The Local Public Health System Assessment	Measures the capacity of the local public health system to conduct essential public health services
The Community Health Status Assessment	Analyzes data about health status, quality of life, and risk factors in the community
The Forces of Change Assessment	Identifies forces that are occurring or will occur that affect the community or local public health system

After deciding what to scan, the process moves to the next step, monitoring.

Monitoring. Effectively scanning the external environment of a program or project identifies and organizes specific information about trends, developments, and events that represent either opportunities or threats for continued attention through monitoring. Monitoring is more than scanning. It involves tracking or following important information over time.

Aspects of the external environment are monitored or tracked because they are thought to be of relevance to the program or project's future. Monitoring these aspects of the environment, especially when there is ambiguity as to their importance to the future, permits more information to be assembled about trends, developments, and events to clarify their importance or determine the rate at which they may be becoming important to the program or project's future.

Monitoring has a much narrower focus than scanning because the purpose in monitoring is to build a base of data and information around the set of important or potentially important aspects of the external environment that were identified through scanning or verified through earlier monitoring. Usually far fewer aspects of a program or project's external environment are monitored than are scanned.

Monitoring is extremely important because it is so often difficult to determine whether information about trends, developments, or events actually represents either real opportunities or threats for a program or project. Under conditions of certainty, managers would fully understand the information and all its consequences for their decisions and actions. However, uncertainty characterizes much about the external environments of programs and projects and uncertainty cannot be removed completely. Uncertainty can, however, be significantly reduced by the acquisition of more detailed and sustained information through effective monitoring. As with scanning, techniques that feature the acquisition of multiple perspectives and expert opinions can be helpful. Careful monitoring and tracking provides the background for the next step in analyzing a program or project's external environment, forecasting changes in the external environment.

Forecasting. Scanning and monitoring cannot, in and of themselves, provide managers with all the information they need about their program or project's external environment. Often, if they are to use this information effectively in strategizing, they need *forecasts* of future conditions or states. This may give them time to adjust desired results or formulate and implement successful operational plans in response to the new conditions.

Scanning and monitoring external environments involves searching for early signals that may be the forerunners of what will become strategically important information about trends, developments, and events. Forecasting involves extending information beyond its current state.

Forecasts of some types of information can be made by extending past trends or by applying a formula of some kind. In other situations, forecasting must rely upon conjecture, speculation, and judgment. Sometimes even sophisticated simulations can be conducted to forecast the future. However, uncertainty characterizes the results of all these methods. It is especially difficult to include in any of these approaches the fact that few strategically important pieces of information exist in a vacuum. Many different pieces of information must be considered simultaneously. Many variables work together simultaneously, and no forecasting techniques or models have been developed to fully account for this fact.

A widely used forecasting technique is *trend extrapolation.* When properly used, this technique can be remarkably effective and it is relatively simple to use. Trend extrapolation is nothing more than tracking information and then using the tracking results to predict future states. It works best to predict general trends, such as the number of patients/customers who will be served by a program or its reimbursement rate for certain services from Medicare or Medicaid. For example, if the number of patients/customers has increased by 5 percent for each of the past five years, it may be reasonable to assume a 5 percent increase in the next year.

Another useful forecasting technique is *scenario development.* A scenario is a plausible prediction about the future. This technique is especially appropriate for analyzing environments that include many uncertainties and imponderables, such as the external environments many health programs and projects face.

The essence of scenario development is to define several alternative future states. These predictions can be used as the basis for developing contingency plans; alternatively, the set of scenarios can be used to select what a manager considers the most likely future, the one upon which strategizing the future will be based.

Multiple scenarios permit several future possibilities to be explored. After a range of possibilities has been reflected in a set of scenarios, managers may choose one to be the most likely scenario if they wish. However, a common mistake in using scenario development is to envision too early in the process one particular scenario as the correct picture of the future.

Assessing. Scanning and monitoring information that is relevant to strategizing the future and making accurate forecasts of trends in the information are each important steps in conducting an external environmental analysis. However, managers must also concern themselves about the specific and relative strategic importance of the information they are analyzing. That is, they must *assess* the strategic importance and implications of the acquired information and forecasts for their programs or projects.

Making these assessments is not an exact science. More than anything else, it relies upon the judgment of the people making the assessments. Even so, there are several bases upon which the strategic importance of information in an external environment can be considered. Prior experience with similar information is frequently a useful basis for assessing the importance of information.

Other bases include intuition or best guesses about what particular information might mean to a program or project, as well as advice and insight from others who are well-informed and experienced. When possible, quantification, modeling, and simulation of the potential impact can be useful, but this is often beyond the resources of a program or project.

It is rarely a simple task to accurately determine the information's relevance and importance to the future of a program or project. Aside from the difficulties encountered in collecting and properly analyzing enough information to fully inform the assessment, there sometimes are problems that derive from the influence of the personal preferences and biases of those conducting the environmental analysis. Such problems can force assessments that fit preconceived notions about what is strategically important rather than reflecting the realities of the impact of particular information. As with other steps in the external situational analysis, obtaining multiple judgments about the strategic importance of information can help avoid the bias problem.

Using and Disseminating. The final step in analyzing a program or project's external situation involves *using* the acquired information and forecasts in strategizing, which may include *disseminating* or spreading the information to all those whose decisions and actions might be affected by it. This step is frequently undervalued as part of the conduct of an external environmental assessment; it may even be overlooked. Unless information is disseminated to and used by all who need it, however, it does not matter how well the other steps in the assessment are performed.

Managers must base their strategizing on valid information about their program or project's external environment if this core activity is to be properly performed. In many cases, managers need to share the information with others as well. For example, in a large program or project, there may be sub-divisions with managers of their own who must engage in strategizing activity. Managers can disseminate the strategically important information obtained through the conduct of an environmental analysis in the following three ways:

- Dictate or require use of the information, perhaps using coercion or sanctions to see that the information is used in all the appropriate places in the program or project.
- Persuade others to use the information by reasoning with them.
- Educate others as to the importance and usefulness of the information in their own strategizing activities.

In dictating use, managers simply rely on the power associated with their position to dictate that the information is to be used. Other participants in the program or project are expected to carry out the dictates by using the information in their own strategizing. Such dictates have appropriate uses. For example, an abrupt and surprising change in a state's reimbursement policy for Medicaid services might require an immediate shift in how a program operates, leaving little time for anything but an edict to ensure the use of this information in revising an operational plan.

Dictates have the advantage of being fast and easy for managers to issue, although a major drawback is their disruptiveness and recipients' feelings of nonparticipation in the conduct of the environmental assessment.

The more participative persuasion and education approaches work better when time permits their use. These approaches are greatly facilitated when those who will end up using the information from an external environmental assessment participate in its production. Participation can be achieved through such devices as membership on committees or teams charged to conduct the scanning, monitoring, forecasting, and assessing aspects of the assessment.

Using and disseminating the strategically important information about a program or project's external environment brings the process of analyzing that external environment to completion. The level of comfort any program or project feels about its external environment depends very heavily on the quality with which the external environmental assessment is conducted. However, this is only the first half of a complete situational analysis. An external environmental assessment only partially answers the question "How are we situated now?" A complete answer also requires information about the internal situation of a program or project.

Internal Situational Analysis

The second part of conducting a situational analysis is an internal analysis, which involves cataloguing both the strengths and weaknesses inherent in a program or project. This analysis provides managers with an inventory of the program or project's resource base for use in strategizing the future. To ensure a systematic inventory, a framework should guide the analysis, including at least the following components:

- A financial analysis covering the program or project's financial condition, trends in its financial performance, revenue streams, and funding sources; this may include how a program or project compares to industry norms or to similar programs or projects.
- A human resources analysis covering the program or project's capabilities to perform its direct, support, and management work. This analysis should provide information on the adequacy of participants in terms of numbers and

credentials, both for present activities and for possible future development. This analysis sometimes covers cultural aspects of the participants in a program or project. Cultural aspects include shared beliefs (such as the centrality of patient care, the importance of medical research, the primacy of quality in health services delivery) and shared values (such as duty, integrity, trust, and fairness). Cultural aspects help guide the behavior of participants. While this part of a human resources analysis may involve a degree of subjectivity, it can be an important component of a complete internal resource analysis.

- A marketing analysis covering all aspects of the program or project's ability to distribute its services. This analysis should identify the program or project's markets and its competitive position (market share) within these markets.

- An operations analysis covering the program or project's various production or service delivery activities. This analysis should cover activities in the direct work of the program or project, but it should also cover support and management operations as well. In terms of the program or project's logic model, this analysis focuses on the processes component of Figure 1.1.

Inventory of Desired Results

The third component of a complete situational analysis is an inventory of the desired results established for a program or project. These should exist as written statements of the desired outputs, outcomes, and impact that have been established for a program or project. Most programs and large projects should also have written *mission statements*. If there is a mission statement, it should also be included in the inventory.

Typically, a mission statement is a broad, general expression of a program or project's overall purpose or purposes. For example, the University of Pittsburgh Medical Center (UPMC) has embedded within it a large program in community health. The expressed mission of this program is "to utilize the collective resources of UPMC, including those of the University of Pittsburgh Schools of the Health Sciences, to improve the health status of the communities in its service area" (http://www.upmc.com). This statement contains the key elements of a useful mission statement, which include what a program or project intends to do and for whom. The degree to which this program accomplishes its mission determines much about its impact.

As shown in Figure 1.1, a program or project's impact is the ultimate change it causes to occur. Impact is the degree to which a program or project's mission is accomplished. If the UPMC's program in community health achieves its mission, the program's impact will be improved health status in the communities in its service area. Like the mission statement of UPMC's program in community health, mission statements tend to be qualitative. For example, the mission of the Breast Cancer Program of the Dana-Farber-Harvard Cancer Center is "to reduce death due to breast cancer and to lengthen and improve the quality of life of women with this disease" (http://www.dfhcc.harvard.edu/dfhcc/ breastcancer.htm). If this program's mission is accomplished, the program's impact will be reduced death from breast cancer and longer and improved quality of life for women with this disease. However, the statement does not specify how many deaths will be avoided or how much the quality of life for women with breast cancer will be improved.

Although most mission statements are inherently qualitative, others incorporate more precise quantitative terms. For example, the San Francisco Immunization Coalition is a program made up of diverse public and private members whose mission is "to achieve and maintain full immunization protection for each child in San Francisco in order to promote community health and wellness" (http://www.dph.sf.ca.us/HealthInfo/SFIC/ImmunizeCoalition.htm). If this mission were fully accomplished, every child in San Francisco would have full immunization protection and the community would enjoy more health and wellness.

Mission statements and desired impacts are important expressions of what programs and projects intend to accomplish. However, they are usually too general to fully guide the work done in programs and projects. Thus, the more concrete statements of desired outputs and outcomes are very important.

Both outputs and outcomes express the specific results a program or project seeks to accomplish. Outputs pertain to the direct results of a program or project's operation and are often expressed in the form of numbers and types of services provided. Outcomes are expressions of changes in the patients/ customers served by a program or project or changes in the operation of the program or project that are desired. Outcomes reflect changes in the behavior, knowledge, health status, or level of functioning caused in the patients/customers served by a program or project. Outcomes can also be expressed as desired changes in some aspect of the program or project's resources and inputs, and also as changes in its processes. For example, a program can establish an outcome statement to express the desire to attain a quality level consistent with best practice guidelines or to have all patients/customers treated in a culturally sensitive manner.

Statements of both desired outputs and outcomes should, to the extent possible, be concrete and specific. This means they should be quantifiable and related to a time frame. For example, a desired output expressed as 100 units of a service provided in a six-month period is more useful as a guide to action than an expression of the desired output to achieve 100 units of a service with no time frame specified. Statements of desired outputs and outcomes should be realistic, achievable, and understandable to the participants in a program or project who are responsible for their accomplishment.

Quantifying desired outputs and outcomes allows people to pinpoint their accomplishments. Every participant in a program or project who has responsibility for specific outputs or outcomes and who is provided adequate resources can and should be held accountable for the results. Accountability for accomplishing results is clearer if the results are measurable. This does not mean, however, that quantified statements cannot be changed.

Circumstances change and may necessitate changes to stated desired outputs or outcomes. For example, a program may have established an outcome of holding payroll expenditures for the year below a certain level. However, if the number of patients/customers increases above that which was projected when the outcome statement was developed, then the outcome statement may have to be altered to remain appropriate in the new circumstances.

When mission statements, as well as statements of desired outputs, outcomes, and impact for a program or project do not exist in writing, preparing them becomes a critical task in effective strategizing. These statements are necessary components in conducting a situational analysis to determine the current situation of a program or project. Figure 2.1 provides a template for developing these statements and offers examples of each type of desired result. Note that the template follows the components of a basic logic model as shown in Figure 1.1.

The information collected through conducting the external and internal situational analyses, along with the inventory of desired results for a program or project, provides an answer to the first question in strategizing: What is the current situation of our program or project? This information also serves as the background for answering the second question in strategizing.

In What Ways Do We Want Our Program or Project's Situation to Change in the Future?

Reconsidering and Revising the Logic Model

Using the information obtained in answering the first question in strategizing, a program or project's manager has a starting point for strategizing the program or project's future. In order to establish a blueprint for its future state, a program or project's entire logic model must be reconsidered, and revisions made

FIGURE 2.1. TEMPLATE FOR DEVELOPING DESIRED RESULTS FOR A PROGRAM OR PROJECT.

Inputs/Resources	Processes	Outputs	Outcomes	Impact (degree to which mission is accomplished)
		The direct results of the processes undertaken by a program or project (such as meetings held, reports written, services provided, classes taught, materials produced and distributed)	Changes in attitudes, behaviors, knowledge, health status, level of functioning resulting from the processes undertaken by a program or project (such as 25% increase in follow-up visits; 50 volunteers regularly serve program; 80 people stop smoking; 90% immunization rate achieved; 100 people complete series of diabetes education classes; 20% increase in foundation funding)	Ultimate changes resulting from a program or project (such as improved health status in community; reduced rate of child abuse; lower incidence of new type 2 diabetes cases; patient/customer satisfaction ratings stabilize at 92% for 3 years; new trauma center opens; new satellite clinic facility opens)
		Examples of Statements of Desired Outputs 1. Increase service sessions by 10% 2. Enroll 500 patients/customers 3. Produce new educational brochure 4. Others	**Examples of Statements of Desired Outcomes** 1. 100 pregnant teenagers receive appropriate prenatal care 2. 90% immunization rate achieved 3. All program participants trained in cultural sensitivity 4. Others	**Examples of Statements of Desired Impact** 1. Health status in target neighborhood improves 2. Program achieves sustainable funding 3. Patients receive state-of-the-art cancer care 4. Others

as necessary. Changes can be made in any part of a logic model as managers consider how they want their programs and projects to be situated in the future (usually in the next year, although strategizing can also be done in multi-year increments). It is not unusual, for example, for a program or project to have a five-year plan or strategy.

The San Francisco Immunization Coalition has an existing set of desired outputs, outcomes, and impact that include the following:

- Achieve on-time immunization of 90 percent of children by age two by the year 2010
- Promote and provide appropriate immunization information and education
- Eliminate barriers to immunization
- Effectively use and coordinate the expertise and resources of coalition partners

In answering the question of how this program should be situated in the future (assume the next year), those who are involved in strategizing its future can reconsider and revise these and other statements of desired results. They can add new statements and also delete or modify existing statements as they choose. By reconsidering and revising the statements of desired results, they restate what they intend for the program to accomplish in the future.

The reconsideration and revision necessary in determining a preferred future state for a program or project does not end with changes in statements of desired results. It includes the other components of the logic model as well. Although details of operational plans about how to accomplish changes in the flow of inputs/resources into a program or project, or about how to change the processes it uses, are developed in answering the third question in strategizing (How will we move our program or project to the preferred future state?), attention is given to these components of a program or project's logic model as managers envision a preferred future state for the program or project.

In developing a preferred future state for their programs and projects, managers must consider whether new resources such as additional funding or people with different educational backgrounds and credentials are needed to accomplish new desired results. They might consider possible changes in existing resources, such as redirecting existing funding or retraining existing staff. They must also consider changing existing processes, either by addition, deletion, or modification. These changes can be made in order to accomplish new desired results or to improve the efficiency or quality of work processes intended to attain existing desired results.

Typically, changes in inputs/resources and processes are necessary if new desired results are to be attained. However, such changes may be difficult to make. It is well-documented in health care settings that changes in work processes are difficult to establish and maintain. The inertia built into established patterns of work and the effort necessary to implement new work processes make changing processes very challenging (Pettigrew, Woodman, and Cameron 2001; Ham, Kipping, and McLeod 2003).

Changing the desired results for a program or project can also be difficult. Sometimes managers find it difficult to establish a new desired output or outcome when its selection means giving up a previously established output or outcome. When a decision is made to establish specific desired results or when a decision is made to commit resources to achieve results, other alternatives must then be forgone. Some managers may find it difficult to accept the fact that their program or project cannot achieve all the results that are important to them and may therefore be reluctant to make firm commitments to specific statements of desired results; they want to avoid the painful consequence of giving up pursuit of other desirable results.

Another problem that affects some managers at the point of establishing the desired results for their programs or projects is their concern they might fail to accomplish the intended results. Whenever a manager sets a definite, clear-cut desired result—whether in the form of an output, outcome, or impact—there is an accompanying risk that the result will not or cannot be achieved. Concerns about such failure prevent some managers from establishing definitive statements of desired results against which their performance can eventually be judged. Those who lack confidence in their abilities to attain results or who are highly risk-averse may be reluctant to establish difficult or challenging statements of desire for their programs or projects.

In spite of such difficulties, managers must be explicit in stating desired outputs, outcomes, and impact for their programs and projects if these decisions are to serve as guides in moving to a desired future state. Similarly, managers must consider the resource and process implications of revising the desired results established for their program or project. These decisions, after all, reflect the answer to the question of how they want their program or project to be situated in the future. These decisions also establish the parameters of the challenge of moving the program or project to its new preferred state.

How Will We Move Our Program or Project to the Preferred Future State?

Developing Operational Plans to Accomplish Desired Results

The accomplishment of desired results in a program or project, including moving to a preferred future state, depends upon developing and implementing good *operational plans*. Statements of desired results, whether in the form of outputs, outcomes, or impact, can be thought of as the *ends* toward which those involved in a program or project work; operational plans are the detailed *means* of how the ends can be accomplished.

Once decisions about ends have been made, decisions about means can be addressed. In operational planning, managers develop and assess alternative means for achieving established ends, and select the specific manner in which the ends will be pursued. Much of the day-to-day management work in programs and projects consists of finding effective means to accomplish established ends.

While there is no formula by which the most appropriate means to accomplish ends are selected, once alternative ideas about the means to accomplishing ends have been placed on a menu for consideration, their relative advantages, disadvantages, and potential effects and implications can be assessed. The task is to assess the available alternatives relative to each other and select those thought to give the best chance of accomplishing the desired results.

In some situations, operational planning can influence decisions about ends. A desired output, outcome, or impact established for a program or project that cannot be achieved should be reconsidered. Therefore, although we are discussing ends and means in this order, in reality decisions about each influence the other.

If a manager concludes that a particular statement of a desired result developed in answering the previous question about a program or project's preferred future state cannot be achieved with available or obtainable inputs and processes, then the desired result must be modified or abandoned. Similarly, a manager choosing between two equally attractive ends for a program or project—when both cannot be achieved simultaneously—can readily make the choice if operational planning determines that one attractive end will cost significantly more than another. However, great care must be exercised in permitting assessments of means to influence decisions about ends. In general, means are not as important as ends. Means are but ways to achieve the ends of a program or project. A program or project's ends in the form of outputs, outcomes, and impact are the reason it exists.

Choosing from Alternatives in Developing an Operational Plan

Armed with comparative information based on assessments of alternatives, managers can choose from among their alternatives in an informed way as they develop operational plans. In making such decisions, as with other types of management decisions, selection of the means to accomplish a program or project's ends can be based on experience, intuition, advice from consultants or colleagues, on systematic analyses to identify the alternative that most closely fits a set of criteria, or on some combination of these bases. In making these decisions, managers can also be guided by the information provided in Chapter Five, including decision grids, payoff tables, decision trees, and cost-benefit analysis. The Program Evaluation and Review Technique, PERT, can be especially useful in assessments of the timing of elements in operational plans.

Managers, as they actually choose from among alternatives in developing an operational plan, face some of the same difficulties that all decision makers face at the point of decision. For example, they may hesitate because they are not certain they have assembled all the relevant information. Collecting and analyzing information in the situational analysis is often difficult, and there is the persistent problem of knowing when enough information has been considered to ensure a well-informed planning process. This problem exists in most decision-making circumstances. In addition, managers can be indecisive or impulsive, just as decision makers in other situations can be.

The difficulties inherent in making the choices necessary in formulating operational plans are not insurmountable. Generally, the difficulties are reduced as managers gain experience with operational planning. The value of experience applies equally to managers' efforts to establish realistic statements of desired outputs, outcomes, and impact for their programs or projects. In addition, managers who have the opportunity to receive coaching and counseling from more experienced managers are better able to develop their capabilities in operational planning and to enhance other aspects of their strategizing.

Coaching and counseling can occur quite naturally in programs or projects that are embedded in larger organizations. The manager's immediate superior in the organization can provide training and guidance in establishing statements of desired results and in developing suitable operational plans to achieve results. In addition, recognition and reward for success provided by the superior can reinforce learning, and constructive and supportive critiques of mistakes can provide valuable learning opportunities for less-experienced managers.

Managers who lack confidence in their ability to develop good operational plans can benefit from participating in management development programs. One of the important purposes of these programs is to enhance managers' abilities to make better decisions, including those made within the context of strategizing. When programs or projects are embedded in an organization that provides management development opportunities, that has a well-understood approach to strategizing, and that devotes sufficient resources to the activity, it is easier for all managers to effectively strategize. In the absence of organizational support, managers must seek to develop and enhance their capabilities within the resources of the program or project, or through participation in outside management development opportunities provided through professional associations and universities.

Implementation Considerations in Operational Planning

The development of good operational plans includes careful attention to factors that will affect their implementation, including information on resources, attitudes about the plan, and information about other operational plans being implemented simultaneously. Operational plans, no matter how carefully crafted, do not implement themselves. Attention must be given to the challenges likely to arise in implementing operational plans during their formulation.

When developing a good operational plan, managers must assess how easy it is to implement in the context of a program or project's capabilities. Ideally, managers recognize the connection between plans and implementation capability and factor this into operational planning decisions. When mismatches occur between operational plans and implementation capabilities, problems invariably arise in their implementation. Such mismatches can be overcome in two ways: plans can be changed, and the capabilities of a program or project to implement a particular operational plan can be changed. In the latter case, resources can be redirected; participants can be provided with additional training and education, and new participants can be brought into the situation to support implementation.

Even when there is a close match between operational plans and implementation capabilities, implementation requires that managers also be effective at designing and leading. Creating organization designs and attracting and retaining participants with the skills and abilities needed to implement operational plans is crucial to the successful implementation of plans. Similarly, leading other participants in playing their parts in successful implementation is also vital.

When a program or project's manager has answered the first three questions in strategizing and knows the current situation thoroughly, has a clear vision of where the program or project should be situated in the future, and has developed operational plans capable of moving to the new state, a fourth question arises as efforts are made to move to the new desired state.

Are We Making Acceptable Progress Toward the Desired Future State?

Assessing Progress and Controlling Performance

The strategizing activity in management work is brought to full circle through a determination of whether or not acceptable progress is being made toward achieving a program or project's desired outputs, outcomes, and impact. By determining whether ongoing performance is acceptable and whether appropriate progress is being made toward achievement of the desired future state established for a program or project, and by making adjustments and corrections if inadequacies are detected, managers increase the likelihood of eventual achievement of the desired results.

Technically, *controlling* in work situations is the regulation of actions and decisions in accord with the stated desired results and with the standards of performance established in operational plans. The word *control* often carries a negative connotation. People sometimes tend to think of it as a sinister activity involving surveillance, correction, or even reproach. But control is a normal part of most human endeavors.

Monitoring the results accomplished and feeding this information back to those who can influence future results is a normal, pervasive, and natural phenomenon in work settings, including health programs and projects. Chefs watch their Hollandaise sauces carefully, DJ's listen to their music, nurses monitor the condition of patients in their care, manufacturers check the quality of products coming off their assembly lines, and soccer coaches watch the scoreboard and clock. All this monitoring is done so that deviations can be detected and corrected in time to favorably affect results.

Controlling, whether expenditures, quality of services, participants' morale, or anything else, involves monitoring performance, comparing actual results with previously established desired results and standards, and correcting deviations that are found. Figure 2.2 illustrates the interrelated parts of controlling performance and assessing progress in the laboratory of a program designed to screen for HIV infection. Note that the work of this laboratory is modeled in terms of the logic model presented in Figure 1.1, with the added elements necessary for assessing progress and controlling performance.

In this model, desired results are those established earlier in strategizing for this program's laboratory. Desired results in the form of outputs, outcomes, and impact are, in effect, the targets or ends desired for a program or project, or, as in this case, a unit of a specific program. Standards are typically those established by professions, regulators, and accrediting agencies. Together, the desired results and the standards become the criteria against which performance can be compared and judged.

To be most useful in controlling, both desired results and standards should be expressed in terms that actual performance can be measured against. Examples include quantity, cost, time, attitude, or quality measures. Controlling is facilitated when the criteria against which performance will be assessed are expressed in objective terms, although this works better in some situations than in others. For example, a desired outcome of a high level of participant morale may be more difficult to specify in objective terms than a desired outcome of successfully operating within an established budget in a given year. However, it is possible to devise and use methods of subjectively determining whether movement is toward or away from achievement of a desired outcome of improved morale.

FIGURE 2.2. CONTROL OF PERFORMANCE IN AN HIV-SCREENING PROGRAM'S LABORATORY.

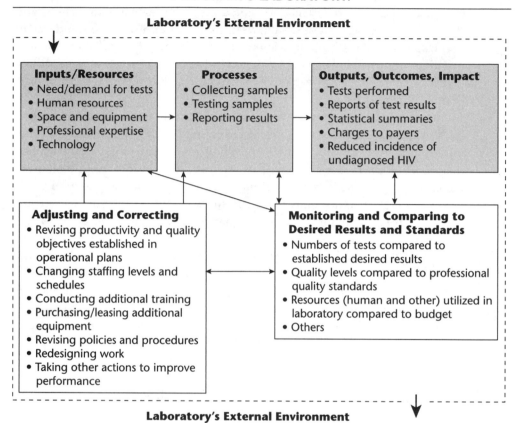

Laboratory's External Environment

Inputs/Resources
- Need/demand for tests
- Human resources
- Space and equipment
- Professional expertise
- Technology

Processes
- Collecting samples
- Testing samples
- Reporting results

Outputs, Outcomes, Impact
- Tests performed
- Reports of test results
- Statistical summaries
- Charges to payers
- Reduced incidence of undiagnosed HIV

Adjusting and Correcting
- Revising productivity and quality objectives established in operational plans
- Changing staffing levels and schedules
- Conducting additional training
- Purchasing/leasing additional equipment
- Revising policies and procedures
- Redesigning work
- Taking other actions to improve performance

Monitoring and Comparing to Desired Results and Standards
- Numbers of tests compared to established desired results
- Quality levels compared to professional quality standards
- Resources (human and other) utilized in laboratory compared to budget
- Others

Laboratory's External Environment

In monitoring and comparing, actual performance is measured. There is no substitute for direct observation and personal contact by managers as they monitor performance, although such techniques are inefficient. Thus, some monitoring is typically done through other means. Written reports on performance can be especially useful for managers with large or diverse domains of responsibility. To monitor performance in large programs or projects, managers may have to rely almost exclusively on written or verbal reports provided by others. In some instances, managers prefer to receive performance reports only when established desired results or standards are not being met, relying on what is called the *exception approach* to monitoring.

Program or project managers also may find information systems (IS) useful in their controlling efforts (Austin and Boxerman 2003). These systems can be designed so that information relevant to control can be collected, formatted, stored, and retrieved in a timely way to support the monitoring and comparing aspects of controlling. An IS can be relatively simple or very elaborate. If it is to be useful, however, an IS should report deviations at critical points. Effective control requires attention to those factors that actually affect a program or project's performance. A good IS will report deviations promptly and contain elements of information that are understandable to those who use the system. Finally, a good IS will point to corrective action. A control system that detects deviations from accomplishment of desired results or from standards will be little more than an interesting exercise if it does not show the way to corrective action. A good IS will disclose where failures are occurring and who is responsible for them, so that corrective action can be undertaken.

When monitoring and comparing reveals deviations from the accomplishment of desired results or from adherence to chosen standards, adjustments should be made or corrective actions should be taken. These corrective actions curb undesirable results and bring performance back in line. When deviations occur, effective control requires that corrective actions be taken, as shown in Figure 2.2. However, knowing what actions to take can be a difficult challenge for managers.

Because so many underlying factors can be involved, it is often difficult to determine the flaws in operational plans or why implementation falters. Are the established desired results reasonable? Are the operational plans adequate? Is the implementation of operational plans going smoothly? Are there adequate resources, and are participants properly trained to implement the operational plan?

Managers should base their decisions about adjustments and corrective actions on a careful analysis of the situation, starting with consideration of the desired results and standards against which they are monitoring performance. After all, the desired results may have been poorly conceived, or conditions may have changed, rendering them inappropriate. Too, standards undergo revisions from time to time. When standards are changed, adjustments may be necessary in resources or processes being used.

Only after a thorough analysis of the reasons for a deviation will a manager be in a position to take effective corrective action that will secure improved results in the future. Such corrective action may consist of revising desired results, changing a process, redeploying resources, having a simple discussion with participants about their work, employing a change in technology, increasing training, improving equipment, budgeting more time, creating a new schedule, or doing anything else to rectify the situation. Armed with an understanding of the causes of deviations, managers can undertake effective corrective action. In doing this, they become *change agents*.

Budgets and Effective Control

Managers need effective *control systems* or techniques to support their assessment of progress toward achieving their programs' or projects' missions and objectives, in detecting discrepancies between objectives and actual performance, and in taking corrective action. In their efforts to control performance, health programs and projects routinely develop *budgets*, which are the most widely used type of control system.

Budgets reflect projected activities of programs, projects, or subunits within a program or project in numerical terms covering a specified period of time. Their use as control systems derives from the fact that budgets are used as pre-established objectives or standards against which actual operating results can be compared and adjusted through the exercise of control.

Budgets provide information that enables managers to take corrective action when necessary to bring results into conformity with targets. Although budgets often are expressed in monetary terms, they can be expressed in other units as well. Personnel budgets, for example, indicate the number of people needed at various skill levels and the number of person-hours allocated for certain activities.

For most programs and projects, an *operating budget*, which is a combination of a *revenue budget* and an *expense budget*, may be the only budget required for controlling purposes. Exhibit 2.1 contains the annual operating budget for a large program designed to provide a range of health services on a fee-for-service (FFS) basis to patients/customers who use the program. The program also provides services to an enrolled population that includes 12,000 members. These services are provided under contract on a capitated or pre-paid basis.

The construction of an operating budget for this program requires volume projections or estimates as a starting point. Based on past experience, the manager estimates that 20,000 visits to the program will be made by FFS patients/customers in Year X. In addition, the capitated population has averaged 0.20 visits per member-month. Therefore, the manager calculates that in Year X the capitated population will produce $12,000 \times 12 = 144,000$ member-months. The manager uses the historical average of 0.20 visits per member-month to calculate an estimated number of visits by the capitated population as follows: $144,000 \times 0.20 = 28,800$ visits. Estimated total volume expressed as the number of visits to the program for services for Year X is $20,000 + 28,800 = 48,800$ visits. (These volume assumptions are shown as Part I in Exhibit 2.1)

EXHIBIT 2.1. A PROGRAM'S OPERATING BUDGET FOR YEAR X.

Part I   Volume Assumptions

A.	Fee-for-service (FFS)	20,000	visits

B.	Capitated lives (plan members)	12,000	members
	Number of member-months	144,000	
	Expected utilization per member-month	0.20	visits
	Number of visits	28,800	visits

C.	Total expected visits	48,800	visits

Part II   Revenue Assumptions

A.	FFS	$ 40	per visit
		× 20,000	visits
		$ 800,000	

B.	Capitated lives	$ 4	per member per month
		× 144,000	member-months
		$ 576,000	

C.	Total expected revenues	$1,376,000	

Part III   Cost Assumptions

A.	Variable costs		
	Staffing (26,000 hours @ $28 per hour)	$ 728,000	
	Supplies	90,000	
	Total variable costs	$ 818,000	
	Variable cost per visit	$ 16.76	($818,000/48,800 visits)

B.	Fixed costs		
	Overhead, depreciation, leasing	$ 400,000	

C.	Total expected costs	$1,218,000	

Part IV Pro Forma Profit and Loss (P&L) Statement

Revenues		
FFS	$800,000	
Capitated	576,000	
Total	$1,376,000	
Variable costs	$ 818,000	
Contribution margin	558,000	($1,376,000-$818,000)
Fixed costs	400,000	
Projected profit	$ 158,000	

To calculate the revenue budget, the manager assumes the program's net collection for the FFS visits will average $40 per visit. Some visits will produce more revenue, some less. On average, however, past experience yields an estimate of $40 per visit from the FFS patients/customers. Thus, FFS revenues would be estimated as 20,000 visits × $40 = $800,000 for 2006. Using the contract premium established for the capitated population of $4 per member per month (PMPM), the manager can calculate revenue from this source as $4 × 144,000 member-months = $576,000 for Year X. Combining FFS and capitated patients/customers, the manager can estimate total revenue for the program in Year X as $800,000 + $576,000 = $1,376,000. These revenue assumptions are shown as Part II in Exhibit 2.1. It should be emphasized that this is an estimate of the program's revenues; conditions could change, making the estimate inaccurate.

Part III of the operating budget shown in Exhibit 2.1 contains information on the program's estimated expenses for Year X. The manager, again relying upon past experience with the program's operations, estimates that the anticipated 48,800 visits will require a combined staffing cost of $14.92 per visit. This includes staff involved in direct, support, and management work in the program, and is calculated as follows: 26,000 hours of estimated staff time × $28 per hour on average = $728,000. Thus, staff costs per visit are expected to average $728,000/48,800 = $14.92. Although not all costs for staff doing direct and support work are variable as shown in Exhibit 2.1, the use of part-time staff and the payment of some staff on the basis of productivity permits the manager to closely tie the number of hours of estimated staff time to the number of estimated visits.

The other portion of estimated expenses is for supplies. The manager estimates that medical and administrative supplies will cost $90,000 in Year X, based on past patterns of these expenses and the estimated volume of activity. This means that supply costs will average $1.84 per visit ($90,000/48,800 visits). Thus, the program's combined staffing and supplies costs per visit in Year X are estimated to be $14.92 + $1.84 = $16.76.

Finally, as can be seen in Part III of Exhibit 2.1, the program is expected to incur $400,000 of fixed costs in Year X. These expenses include overhead costs, as well as depreciation of equipment and the cost of leasing the program's space to serve the program's anticipated 48,800 visits by its patients/customers in Year X. Variable costs are expected to total $818,000 ($728,000 in staffing and $90,000 in supplies), plus $400,000 in fixed costs, for a total of $1,218,000.

Part IV of Exhibit 2.1 shows the determination of the program's *pro forma* (projected) profit and loss (P&L) statement. The P&L statement is the heart of an operating budget. The difference between projected revenues of $1,376,000 and projected variable costs of $818,000 produces a total contribution margin of

$558,000. Deducting the forecasted fixed costs of $400,000 yields a budgeted profit for the program of $158,000.

Budgets are merely guides for managers, not substitutes for good judgment. Effective budgets allow managers the necessary latitude and flexibility to accomplish the objectives established for their programs and projects when conditions change within the period covered by the budgets. To avoid having budgets become too restrictive, enlightened managers assure flexibility in the use of budgets by monitoring operating conditions and revising budgets when conditions appreciably change. Additional information on budgeting can be found in Gapenski (2002) and Nowicki (2001).

The Link Between Strategizing and the Performance of Programs and Projects

Effective strategizing is crucial to the overall performance of programs and projects. The contribution it makes to performance begins with the focus on desired results that good strategizing requires. Strategizing yields appropriate statements of desired outputs, outcomes, and impact, and it supports managers in developing operational plans for accomplishing the desired ends. In this way strategizing contributes to focusing on desired ends and coordinating the use of a program or project's inputs and resources toward achieving the desired ends.

Strategizing also contributes to performance by helping managers to at least partially offset the effects of pervasive uncertainty. When managers think about the future in systematic ways and plan for contingencies, they greatly reduce the chances of being caught unprepared.

Through the development of operational plans and through assessing and controlling performance, managers also enhance operational efficiency and effectiveness. As noted in Chapter One, strategizing substitutes integrated effort in place of random activity, controlled flow of work in place of uneven flow, and careful decisions in place of snap judgments. These and other results of effective strategizing contribute directly to operational efficiencies in programs and projects and to the effectiveness of direct, support, and management work.

Finally and ultimately most importantly, effective strategizing facilitates the continual assessment of progress toward accomplishment of the desired results established for a program or project, and the exercise of control over the performance of direct, support, and management work in pursuit of these ends. This is increasingly important as those who pay for the services provided through health programs and projects—indeed, all health services—whether through public programs such as Medicare and Medicaid or private employers and their insurance mechanisms, require greater accountability from those who provide these services.

The required accountability goes beyond cost to include both the quality of services and the manner in which they are delivered. The trend toward more accountability and the concurrent need to control ensure that accountability will become increasingly important in all health services settings. Its relationship to managers' efforts to control performance for which they are responsible is one of the most important reasons for effective strategizing in health programs and projects.

Before concluding this chapter, two topics related to strategizing will be covered, *initial strategizing* and *interventional planning*. The unique circumstances of the initial strategizing for a program or project as it is being conceived are discussed in terms of developing a *business plan*. Interventional planning, which is the application of planning techniques to the development, implementation, and evaluation of the interventions that many programs and plans undertake, is also discussed. Interventional planning is undertaken in order to address one or more health determinants that affect the patients/customers a program or project serves. Interventional planning differs from the core strategizing activity that a manager carries out in relation to a program or project. Even so, the success of most interventions or initiatives that a program or project might undertake depends heavily upon effective interventional planning.

Business Plans

One of the most important stages in the life of any program or project is its original conceptualization and then development into a concrete, well-formed idea. At this beginning point, a program or project may be nothing more than an idea or a concept in the imagination of someone who thinks it can meet a real need. An early task in the life of any program or project is for those who support it to demonstrate that the idea is viable. Thus, an initial round of strategizing for a program or project is required. This is termed *business planning* and results in a document called a *business plan* (Abrams 2000).

The concept of business plans emerged in the entrepreneurial world where people with ideas for new businesses must make convincing cases to banks, venture capitalists, and other potential investors in order to attract the necessary capital to get their business to an operational stage. The business plan in these contexts is a written document describing the nature of the business and how the entrepreneur intends to start and operate the business.

The U.S. Small Business Administration, a federal agency that supports the establishment and operation of small business in the United States, notes that a business plan "precisely defines your business, identifies your goals and serves as your firm's resume" (http://www.sba.gov). Because business planning is so ubiquitous, there are many consulting firms—such as Bullet Proof Business Plans (http://www.bulletproofbizplans.com)—available to assist in the process.

A business plan for a nascent health program or project is developed as a means of making a convincing case to all those who must approve its initiation. If a program or project is to be embedded in a larger organization, the audience for the business plan will be organizational superiors who must approve the program or project's initiation.

Although business plans vary in content, a useful business plan for a new health program or project can be constructed around its initial logic model (see Figure 1.1). Development of the logic model provides an opportunity to identify the desired results of the program or project in terms of outputs, outcomes, and impact. It also provides an opportunity to identify the inputs and resources and the various processes that will yield the anticipated results. In addition to the logic model, several other elements are typically included in a business plan, including the following:

- A summary description of the program or project, including summary statements about the elements of the logic model (such as inputs/resources, processes, outputs, outcomes, and impact)
- An explanation of why the program or project is needed and why it will succeed in its market
- A description of the target markets for the program or project, with projections of need and demand for its services, and, as appropriate, projections of sales and market share for the first five years of operation
- A description of how the program or project will be managed, including information on the qualifications of key participants involved
- A description of how the clinical services (if applicable) of the program or project will be provided, including information on the qualifications of key participants involved
- A detailed operating budget, usually projected for the first year of the new program or project and also projected through the first five years of operation (discussed in previous section about preparation of operating budgets)
- A detailed description of space and equipment needed for the first five years of operation
- A description of funding sources for the program or project, including revenues expected from operations, grants, contracts, and other sources of funding

- An analysis of the major risks or challenges faced by the program or project in its first five years, and a description of how these will be addressed
- A timetable of key events and accomplishments expected for the program or project in its first five years

Comprehensive business plans for new programs and projects cannot guarantee their success. They can, however, assure that careful thought is given to the early operational phase of a program or project and to preparing to meet the challenges that can be seen in this special form of strategizing its future.

Planning for Interventions Undertaken by Programs and Projects

Within the overall strategizing activities—through which managers, perhaps with the involvement of others, determine the desired results for programs and projects and develop detailed operational plans for how they will be accomplished—is another form of planning. This form of planning, which we will call *interventional planning,* involves the application of planning techniques to the development, implementation, and evaluation of interventions undertaken by programs and projects as part of their direct work.

In small, highly focused programs or projects—those intended to engage in a single specific intervention such as conducting a single highly focused health education program for example—the distinction between overall strategizing and interventional planning, especially distinguishing between operational planning and interventional planning, may not be possible or relevant. That said, in larger programs and projects there is an important distinction between the overall strategizing done for an entire program or project and the interventional planning done for specific interventions developed and provided within a program or project. An example will help distinguish interventional planning from the more general strategizing activities in which program and project managers engage.

A successful health education program, established by and embedded in a county health department, has served a number of clients for several years. Among the clients are groups of citizens of the county who have been categorized by demographic characteristics (elderly, minority, female teenagers), clinical condition (diabetes, obesity, drug abuse), and affiliation (elementary school students, elderly day-care program participants). All of the health education interventions for these clients are paid for through public funds made available to the health department or through grants from foundations.

In strategizing this program's future, its manager determined it is important to enhance the resources available to the program by adding private, paying clients. The manager envisions many benefits available to the program from broadening the base of financial support through the addition of corporate clients who will pay for services.

In the previous year, the *operational planning* as to how to accomplish this outcome led to some of the program's health educators visiting the benefits managers at local companies and other businesses to explain the advantages of sponsoring various health education interventions for their employees. This resulted in two new clients for the coming year, a large financial services firm and the local plant of an international manufacturing firm.

Good *strategizing* paid off for this health education program, but the success achieved by adding the new clients triggered the need for *interventional planning*. The program manager assigned a health educator to each of the new corporate clients to do the necessary interventional planning to guide the provision of health education services. Interventional planning is undertaken in a series of six steps as shown in Figure 2.3. The health educator's role in each step in the interventional planning for the client is described next.

Figure 2.3. Model of Interventional Planning.

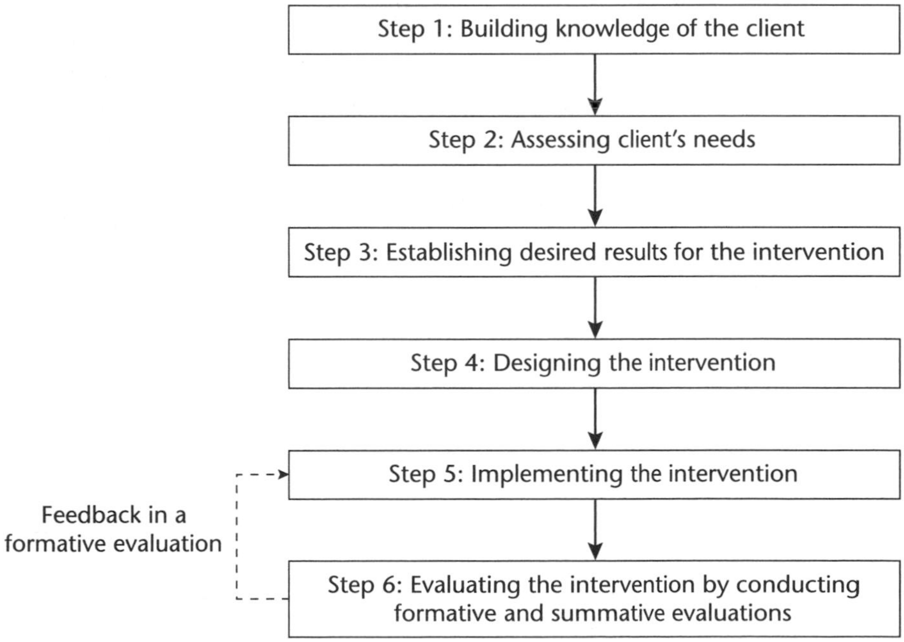

Step 1.   Building knowledge of the client (which can be an organization or
group of individual patients/customers)

Each health educator met separately with a key representative of the new client
to which he had been assigned. For example, one health educator met with the
benefits manager at the plant and with the vice president of human resources
at the financial services company. These meetings were held in order to obtain
the views of these client representatives as to what the intervention might accomplish. In each case, information about the organization, including how employees and their family members use health benefits, was reviewed. Later, in
building knowledge of the client, interviews with groups of employees and family members were conducted. A health education committee was formed with
representation of management and other employees for each client.

Step 2.   Assessing the client's needs for health education

In each situation, with the help of the health education committee, the educator conducted a *needs assessment* (Petersen and Alexander 2001), including a survey of behavioral risk factors that sample groups of employees and their family
members completed. The risk assessment also included several focus group meetings to explore possible needs upon which to focus the intervention. The committees also reviewed insurance claims data for their firm's employees and their
dependents over several years and the Health Plan Employer Data and Information Set (HEDIS), made available by the National Committee on Quality Assurance (NCQA). Data was available for all of the health plans in which
employees and their families were enrolled. (Information is available on NCQA
and HEDIS at http://www.ncqa.org.)

The assessment in both situations identified several areas of need for a health
education intervention. In the financial services company, the most compelling
need was that employees and their adult family members were experiencing a significantly higher rate of type 2 diabetes than would be expected in a population
of this age and gender structure. In the plant, the most compelling problem was
injury prevention among employees, especially back injuries caused by lifting.

Step 3.   Establishing desired results for the intervention

With the involvement of the health education committees, the educators developed statements of the desired results of the interventions. These included impact, as well as more specific results expressed as desired outputs and outcomes.
At the financial services company, the desired impact was to eventually reduce
the incidence of type 2 diabetes among employees and their spouses to a level

consistent with that expected in a group with this age and gender structure. The desired impact for the plant was to reduce the incidence of injuries to a rate no greater than the industry average. In both cases, it was anticipated that these ultimate impacts would take many years to achieve and would not occur until well after the intervention had been completed.

Desired outputs developed for the financial services company included a specific number of face-to-face education sessions to expose employees and spouses to information about diabetes; printed information about preventing, diagnosing, and treating the disease was also produced and distributed. Another desired output was to include information about diabetes on the company's Web site. The committee also established a desired outcome that, following the intervention, all employees with type 2 diabetes would have appropriate hemoglobin A1c (HbA_{1c}), lipids (LDL-C), and kidney disease monitoring (microalbuminuria test), as well as annual eye examinations. Appropriate desired outcomes also were established for the health education intervention at the plant, although the financial services company will be used as the example for the remainder of this discussion.

Step 4. Designing the intervention

The educator assigned to the financial services company designed the intervention to include a number of specific education activities. The design was influenced heavily by the recommendations of the National Diabetes Education Program (NDEP), especially those developed in its section on "The Business Community Takes on Diabetes" (http://www.ndep.nih.gov). The NDEP is a partnership of the National Institutes of Health, the Centers for Disease Control and Prevention and more than 200 public and private organizations. Thus, its recommendations are authoritative.

The design of the intervention also was guided by the educator's use of the design features of a number of well-established health education planning models, including the following:

- PRECEDE-PROCEED Model for Health Promotion Planning and Evaluation (Green and Kreuter 1999)
- Model for Health Education Planning (MHEP) (Ross and Mico 1980)
- Multilevel Approach to Community Health (MATCH) (Simons-Morton, Greene, and Gottlieb 1995)
- CDCynergy, a health communication model developed by the Centers for Disease Control and Prevention (Centers for Disease Control and Prevention, 1999a)
- Social Marketing Assessment and Response Tool (SMART) (Neiger 1998)

- Planning, Program Development, and Evaluation Model (PPDEM) (Timmreck 1995)
- Generalized Model for Program Planning (GMPP) (McKenzie and Smeltzer 2001)

Step 5.   Implementing the intervention

The health educator implemented the intervention by carrying out the activities called for in its design, including distributing a diabetes information sheet with all employees' paychecks. Over the course of implementation, this was followed up with additional information sheets in employee pay envelopes about aspects of diabetes. Two articles about diabetes were written for and included in the company newsletter, and information about the disease was featured on the company's Web site. Posters about the disease were used throughout the company to enhance awareness.

Employees and their family members with diabetes received special mailings with information about how to interact effectively with their physicians. They were provided information produced by the National Diabetes Education Program about specific questions to ask their physicians, including: (1) What are my blood sugar, blood pressure, and cholesterol numbers? (2) What should they be? (3) What actions should I take to reach these goals? Employees and their family members were also given wallet cards on which to record and track these numbers.

Step 6.   Evaluating the intervention

All interventions should be evaluated, although the extent of the evaluation can vary depending upon the importance of its results and the available resources. Useful information for conducting evaluations can be found in a comprehensive framework used by the Centers for Disease Control and Prevention to guide evaluations of its programs (Centers for Disease Control and Prevention 1999b). No matter what specific approach to conducting evaluations is taken, an evaluation is an analytical process involving the collection and analysis of data and information that allows managers to improve interventions while they are in progress or to measure the degree to which the desired results are achieved after the intervention's conclusion (Rossi, Lipsey, and Freeman 2003).

Thus, there are two purposes for evaluating interventions, with the fulfillment of each driving the use of somewhat different methodologies. A *formative evaluation* is intended to help *improve* an intervention as it takes place. A *summative evaluation* is intended to prove whether an intervention accomplished the desired results. The health educator determined that both purposes were relevant to evaluating the intervention at the financial services company and undertook both formative and summative evaluations of the intervention.

A formative evaluation is much like the determination of whether or not acceptable progress is being made toward achieving a program or project's desired outputs, outcomes, and impact as part of the more general strategizing activity. In fact, application of the control model shown in Figure 2.2 can help guide the formative evaluation of an intervention. During a formative evaluation questions are asked about results as they are occurring; this means there is still time to make adjustments when results are not as desired. This type of evaluation requires monitoring the progress being made in an intervention and making mid-course corrections as needed to keep the intervention on track.

The health educator, in conducting the formative evaluation of the intervention at the financial services company, used desired results established in Step 3 to determine progress. As is typical of formative evaluation, the focus was on outputs and outcomes, rather than impact. Impact is typically assessed in a summative evaluation of an intervention.

The educator periodically assessed progress toward achieving the outputs established in Step 3 by determining the number of face-to-face education sessions that had been conducted, as well as progress toward producing and distributing printed information about the prevention, diagnosis, and appropriate treatment of type 2 diabetes. The educator also tracked progress toward the desired outcome of having all employees and spouses with the disease receiving appropriate hemoglobin A1c (HbA_{1c}), lipids (LDL-C), and kidney disease monitoring (microalbuminuria tests), as well annual eye examinations, by the conclusion of the intervention.

When progress toward accomplishment of any of the desired outputs or outcomes established for this intervention was inadequate, the health educator made the necessary adjustments. This is shown conceptually in Figure 2.3 as the feedback loop between the evaluation and implementation steps of the model.

Summative evaluations tend to be snapshots reported after the conclusion of an intervention. Their purpose is to prove or document whether or not an intervention worked as intended and perhaps to summarize the lessons learned from making the intervention. Although in many interventions ultimate impact will not be felt until well past the conclusion of the intervention, the health educator conducting the summative evaluation for the intervention at the financial services company was able to evaluate key outcomes of the intervention. Among these, the educator had specific information of the number and proportion of the company's employees and their spouses who had type 2 diabetes who were receiving appropriate hemoglobin A1c (HbA_{1c}), lipids (LDL-C), and kidney disease monitoring (microalbuminuria tests), as well the number and proportion having an eye examination during the period of the intervention.

It would, however, be some years before anyone could determine if the intervention had its ultimate desired impact of reducing the incidence of type 2 diabetes among the employees and their spouses to a level consistent with what would be expected in a group of this age and gender structure.

Both formative and summative evaluations were performed because each served a different purpose. The formative evaluation of the implementation of the intervention involved collection and analysis of data and information that permitted the educator to assess ongoing progress in the conduct of the intervention and to make improvements in its implementation. The results of ongoing formative evaluation, as well as the actions taken by the health educator in response to the results, were reported to the program manager.

The conduct of the summative evaluation of the intervention required the health educator to collect and analyze data and information to determine how well the intervention worked in terms of achieving its desired results—at least to the extent this data and information were available at the time of the summative evaluation. The results of the summative evaluation were reported to the program manager, who also shared the results with the client company. By proving the result of the intervention, a good case was made to conduct further health education interventions for the financial services company.

The conduct of formative and summative evaluations can be very complicated, in which case the use of consultants is very helpful. Generally, however, managers and other participants can conduct evaluations by focusing on progress toward desired outputs and outcomes in formative evaluations, and impacts in summative evaluations. When impacts will not be determined until far into the future, the focus can be on outcomes achieved at the conclusion of the intervention. Whether simple or complex, however, good interventional planning comes full circle with the completion of the evaluation step in Figure 2.3.

Summary

This chapter defines strategizing as the activities through which a manager, perhaps with the involvement of others, establishes the desired results to be achieved through a program or project and develops operational plans for how the results will be accomplished. The discussion of these activities is structured around how managers of health programs and projects seek answers to the following four questions:

1. What is the current situation of our program or project?
2. In what ways do we want our program or project's situation to change in the future?

3. How will we move our program or project to the preferred future state?
4. Are we making acceptable progress toward the desired future state?

The chapter discusses how question one is answered through the conduct of a thorough situational analysis for a program or project. The situational analysis has three components: an inventory of the desired results established for a program or project, as well as internal and external situational analyses of the program or project.

The conduct of an external situational analyses is discussed in terms of its five interrelated steps: (1) scanning to identify relevant information (trends, developments, or possible events that represent either opportunities or threats for the program or project); (2) monitoring or tracking the relevant information identified through scanning; (3) forecasting or projecting the future directions of relevant information; (4) assessing the implications of the information for the program or project; and (5) disseminating the information to those who can use it to guide decisions and actions.

The conduct of internal situational analysis is discussed in terms of a financial analysis, a human resources analysis, a marketing analysis, and an operations analysis. These analyses provide a catalogue of both the strengths and weaknesses inherent in a program or project.

The inventory of desired results established for a program or project is discussed in terms of a mission statement, as well as statements of desired outputs, outcomes, and impact. Figure 2.1 can serve as a template for developing these statements.

The chapter discusses how question number two is answered through reconsideration of the components of a program or project's logic model, including inputs and resources, processes, outputs, outcomes, and impact. The chapter also discusses how revisions in logic models and organization designs serve as the mechanism to answer question number three about a program or project as its manager strategizes its future. Revisions may involve changing any part of a program or project's inputs, processes, and desired results, and may require detailed operational planning to guide the changes.

The discussion of strategizing is brought to full circle by the answer to question number four in determining whether or not acceptable progress is being made toward achieving a program or project's desired outputs, outcomes, and impact. Controlling is described as the regulation of actions and decisions in accord with the stated desired results—in the form of outputs, outcomes, or impact—and the standards of performance established in operational plans. Figure 2.2 provides an applied example of controlling performance. The roles of information systems (IS) and budgets in control are discussed.

The development of a business plan for a program or project at its original conceptualization and development into a concrete, well-formed idea is discussed. The contents of a good business plan are described, including the development of the initial logic model for the program or project.

Interventional planning is described as a form of planning that takes place within the overall strategizing activities of managers. This form of planning involves the application of planning techniques to the development, implementation, and evaluation of interventions undertaken by programs and projects. A six-step model of interventional planning (see Figure 2.3) is presented in this chapter.

Chapter Review Questions

1. Define strategizing and interventional planning. Distinguish between the two.
2. What four questions must a manager answer in strategizing?
3. What are the components of a complete situational analysis for a program or project?
4. What are the steps in conducting an external situational analysis?
5. What should be included in an internal situational analysis?
6. What should be included in an inventory of a program or project's desired results?
7. Discuss the role of controlling in strategizing.
8. Discuss the role of budgets in controlling.
9. What should be included in a business plan?
10. Discuss the steps in interventional planning.

CHAPTER THREE

DESIGNING FOR EFFECTIVENESS

Managers engage in three highly interrelated core activities in doing management work: *strategizing, designing,* and *leading* (see Figure 1.3). Through *designing* activities, the topic of this chapter, managers shape two important aspects of programs and projects. First, through designing activities, managers establish and revise over time the logic models (see Figure 1.1) of their programs and projects. Second, managers establish and revise the intentional patterns of relationships among human and other resources within their programs or projects through designing activities. These patterns of relationships are called organization designs.

Specifically, the patterns of relationships among human and other resources established by managers are *formal* organization designs. This distinction is important because coexisting within formal organization designs are *informal* structures that exist because people working together within formal designs invariably establish relationships and interactions that lie outside the boundaries of the formal structure. All organization designs have both formal aspects, which are developed by managers, and informal aspects that reflect the wishes and preferences of other participants. This chapter considers both formal and informal aspects of organization designs.

Formal organization designs begin with the designation of individual positions. Positions are subsequently *staffed* as individuals are attracted to occupy them. Individual positions are the basic building block of organization designs, although they are typically clustered into teams or work groups. In larger programs or projects, work groups may be clustered into divisions or other units. When this occurs, issues of how the various work groups and clusters of work groups are integrated and coordinated become important design concerns. Depending upon circumstances, designing activities may also involve relating a program or project to a larger organizational home. For example, a program embedded in a county health department must fit within its larger organizational home. A program manager in such a setting may report to a superior in the larger organizational home.

Designing activities are an ongoing part of management work because the logic models and organization designs of programs and projects undergo continuing revision. Designing for effectiveness means creating logic models and structuring the relationships among human and other resources within a program or project in ways that facilitate the accomplishment of the desired results established through strategizing activities. After reading the chapter, the reader should be able to do the following:

- Understand the designing and revising of logic models
- Understand the staffing process as part of designing
- Appreciate the historical roots of key organization design concepts
- Understand the key organization design concepts, including the following:
    Division of work and specialization of workers
    Authority and responsibility relationships
    Clustering or departmentalization
    Span of control
    Coordination
- Distinguish between formal and informal aspects of organization designs

Designing Logic Models

When managers establish the desired results for a program or project expressed as *outputs, outcomes,* and *impact,* designing is already under way. Desired results are an integral component of the logic model for any program or project (see Figure 1.1) and drive much about how the logic model is designed. The other components of logic models are designed to accomplish the desired results established for a program or project. In designing logic models, managers must carefully consider the *processes* through which *inputs/resources* are used to produce outputs, outcomes, and impact.

Designing the Inputs/Resources Component of Logic Models

In designing the *inputs/resources* component of a logic model (see Figure 1.1), attention is given to the human, financial, technological, and organizational inputs necessary for a program or project to achieve its desired results. Depending upon the situation of a particular program or project, it is likely to require a unique package of resources, typically including some mix of human resources in the form of paid staff and volunteers, funding, potential collaborators, technology, organizational or interpersonal networks, physical facilities, equipment, and supplies (W. K. Kellogg Foundation 2001).

Although all of the inputs and resources needed to make a logic model work are important in considering a program or project's design, none is more important than its human resources. As will be discussed more fully, organization designs of programs and projects begin with the designation of individual positions, which can then be clustered into work groups. When programs and projects are embedded in larger organizations, as many are, organization design continues with clustering work groups into departments and other sub-divisions of the organization, and then grouping and arranging the work groups and clusters of work groups into the entire organization. At the highest level of organization design, individual organizations can be further clustered into systems or alliances of organizations (see Figure 3.1).

Managers at the various levels depicted in Figure 3.1 are concerned with different design issues. Assuming a program or project is embedded in a large organizational context such as a health department, an insurance plan, or a

FIGURE 3.1. A HIERARCHY OF ORGANIZATION DESIGNS.

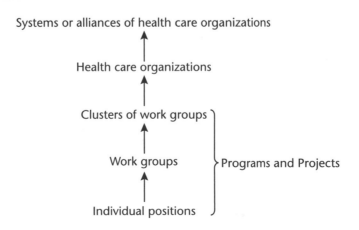

large hospital, top-level managers of the home organization are concerned with design issues such as establishing appropriate relationships between and among work groups and clusters of work groups in the organization. Top-level managers must also search for the synergies that might exist within the organization when all of its parts work together well. They might also be involved in the formation of a system of organizations or with building alliances with other organizations in which their organization is a participating member. In essence, top-level managers are concerned with how effectively the entire organization is designed to achieve the desired results established for it.

Middle-level managers in large organizations are concerned with organizing work groups and clusters of work groups into effective units and divisions. First-level managers in such organizations, however, including those who manage programs or projects within the organization, are directly concerned with establishing and staffing individual positions and with clustering these participants and other resources into the organization design of their program or project. In all organization designs, the fundamental building block is the individual position and the participant who fills the position. Individuals are the starting point from which, through clustering, entire designs are elaborated.

Staffing Health Programs and Projects. Staffing is the process of filling the individual positions established in an organization design with participants. Programs and projects embedded in larger organizations can take advantage of the specially trained human resource professionals who typically orchestrate this highly specialized process in organizations. However, because all managers have staffing responsibilities, the process cannot be left entirely to others.

The staffing process consists of a set of interrelated steps (see Figure 3.2) through which vacant or newly created positions in the organization design are filled. A full discussion of this process is beyond the scope of this book. However, the reader will find excellent, in-depth discussion of general human resource management in Mathis and Jackson (2003); and in Mondy, Noe, Premeaux, and Mondy (2002). Comprehensive discussion of human resource management in health care contexts can be found in Fottler, Hernandez, and Joiner (1998); Fried and Johnson (2002); and Longest, Rakich, and Darr (2000, pp. 531–588). An overview of the steps in the staffing process follows.

The first step in the staffing process, *human resource planning,* involves gathering and analyzing information to identify human resource needs and planning to meet the needs. This planning is influenced by environmental conditions affecting the program or project. It begins with profiling human resource needs at some future date. Short-term (one-year) and long-term (five-year) profiles can be useful. Then the program or project's ability to meet the demands of these profiles can be anticipated and concrete plans for overcoming any shortfalls can be made.

FIGURE 3.2. THE STAFFING PROCESS.

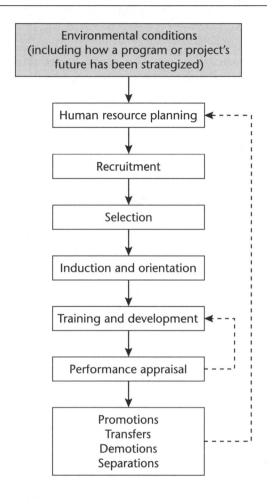

The way a program or project's future has been strategized (see Chapter Two) is very important to its human resource plans. For example, plans to diversify into new activities (such as providing a wellness program) or to significantly increase provision of current services will directly affect the human resource profile. Does the expertise necessary to operate a wellness program exist within the program or project or will new participants need to be recruited? Can current participants be retrained for the new work? And so on. An important part of this planning is maintaining current job descriptions based on careful job analysis for all current and anticipated positions in the program or project.

Guided by the provisions of a human resource plan, *recruitment* of prospective participants is undertaken to develop a pool of job candidates. Candidates are usually attracted through advertisements placed in newspapers and in professional journals, through the efforts of employment agencies, and through visits to educational programs that prepare health professionals. *Selection* involves evaluating and choosing from among job candidates. Application forms, resumes, interviews, and reference checks are standard selection techniques. *Induction and orientation* are activities in the staffing process through which new workers are introduced to their colleagues and to the program or project's history, culture, logic model, and organization design. An important part of this introduction is to thoroughly discuss the desired results established for a program or project and to define the new participant's role in achieving these results. Participants should become acquainted with their responsibilities and be made to feel welcome in their new workplace.

Training and development activities are intended to increase the ability of a program or project's participants to contribute to achieving its desired results. Training usually is specific to current job skills needed by participants; development activities are designed to prepare participants beyond the requirements of their present positions so they can advance or be prepared for new work. Training and development, as illustrated by the feedback loop in Figure 3.2, is partially guided by the results of performance appraisals.

The *performance appraisal* step involves the periodic review and evaluation of the performance of individual participants and, in some cases, the performance of teams. Appraisals serve two purposes, both of which are very important to managing effectively. Appraisals serve an *administrative* purpose in that the information from performance appraisals is taken into account in decisions about compensation, as well as promotions and terminations. Appraisals also serve a *developmental* purpose by identifying strengths and weaknesses among participants, which can be used to guide training and development activities (see the feedback loop in Figure 3.2).

Effective performance appraisal requires that it be based on performance criteria—measurable standards against which performance is compared—that are comprehensive and actually measure aspects of performance that are relevant to the program or project. In the traditional approach to performance appraisal, managers use the performance criteria as a point of comparison while observing actual performance of participants.

Increasingly, however, a broader approach to performance appraisals is employed. This may involve combining a manager's appraisal with a participant's *self-appraisal* of performance. Self-appraisals can be especially useful in tailoring and guiding developmental efforts. An important approach to appraisal in some programs and projects is *team-based appraisal.* In this approach, the performance of a team or group is appraised rather than the performance of a single participant. The major benefit of this approach is that it encourages teamwork; it is especially appropriate when groups or teams of participants work toward achieving specific common outputs, outcomes, and impact, and when any one participant's performance is interdependent with that of other participants in the group.

Originally intended exclusively for developmental purposes, an increasingly popular approach to performance appraisal is the *360-degree appraisal,* also known as a multi-rater assessment or multi-rater feedback. In many settings, 360-degree appraisals are replacing the traditional performance appraisals of individual participants conducted by managers. The central concept of a 360-degree appraisal (and the source of its name) is that an individual's performance can be usefully appraised from many perspectives. (Picture a 360-degree circle of perspectives surrounding the individual.) The raters in this approach can include an individual's organizational superiors, subordinates, peers, patients/customers, and other external stakeholders with whom the participant being appraised has contact. This type of appraisal can serve administrative or developmental purposes, although great care must be exercised in tailoring appraisals for these different uses (Toegel and Conger 2003). Because of its widespread popularity, commercial software for structuring 360-degree appraisals is readily available (for example, http://www.mindsolve.com or http://www.halogensoftware.com), and books on the subject abound (Collins 2000; Lepsinger and Lucia 1997).

The last step in the staffing process is the movement of workers within the program or project through *promotions, demotions,* or *transfers,* and eventually their *separation* from the program or project through resignation, layoff, discharge, or retirement. As the feedback loop in Figure 3.2 illustrates, these movements provide important information for human resource planning.

This overview of staffing is intended to show how the various steps in the process are interrelated. Each of these steps involves very complicated activities, and all aspects of staffing are conducted within a legal context, which includes employment law, labor relations law, and equal employment opportunity law (Fried and Johnson 2002). It is advisable that all program and project managers, when working within the context of a larger organization, use the skills of their organization's human resource department and legal counsel in fulfilling their staffing responsibilities.

It is also advisable that managers pay special attention to diversity among the participants resulting from their staffing efforts. Demographic changes in the United States are creating a more culturally diverse labor pool, as well as a more culturally diverse patient/customer base for programs and projects. Recent studies suggest that cultural diversity is associated with better performance in health care settings (Dansky, Weech-Maldonado, De Souza, and Dreachslin 2003). This derives in part from the relationship between greater diversity and increased *cultural competence,* which supports improved performance.

The Office of Minority Health of the U.S. Department of Health and Human Services has published *National Standards for Culturally and Linguistically Appropriate Services in Health Care* (2001). In this report, cultural competence means "having the capacity to function effectively as an individual or an organization within the context of the cultural beliefs, behaviors and needs presented by consumers and their communities" (p. 131). Among the recommended standards to enhance cultural competence is that all health care organizations—including health programs and projects—should have diverse staffs that are representative of the demographic characteristics of the populations they serve. (See Appendix B, Chapter One, for a description of the project used to develop these standards.)

Designing the Processes Component of Logic Models

In designing the *processes* component of a logic model (see Figure 1.1), attention is given to the activities, events, procedures, and techniques used to perform the direct, support, and management work necessary for a program or project to achieve its desired results. Every program or project, depending upon its specific circumstances, requires a unique mix of processes to achieve its desired results. For example, service provision processes differ in many ways in programs focused on cancer care, cardiac rehabilitation, geriatrics, health education, home care, palliative care, prevention, promotion, research and development, substance abuse, wellness, and women's health. The differences in processes of providing services may be even greater in housing programs, job training programs, or programs intended to clean up the physical environment.

Similarly, significant differences are likely to be found in the processes used in such health projects as research or demonstration projects pertaining to a particular health determinant or in projects to increase seatbelt use, encourage healthier eating, or the practice of safe sex. Other projects—such as those designed to achieve some specific physical or intellectual purpose within a larger program, such as designing and equipping a laboratory, training a staff in a new protocol or how to use a new technology, or designing an information system—may involve even greater differences.

Although many of the processes within programs and projects differ, there are commonalities. For example, many programs and projects share such processes as intake and initial screening of new patients/customers, budget preparation, and interventional planning. An increasingly important and widespread aspect of designing processes in health programs and projects is attention to assuring the *cultural and linguistic appropriateness* of services. As noted previously, the U.S. Department of Health and Human Services, Office of Minority Health, recommends that all programs and projects providing health services ensure that all patients/customers receive from all participants "effective, understandable, and respectful care that is provided in a manner compatible with their cultural health beliefs and practices and preferred language" (2001, p. 49).

Commonalities aside, each program or project is unique in some ways and requires a unique mix of processes if its desired results are to be achieved. Different processes require different activities, events, procedures, and techniques. Depending upon its processes, programs and projects will engage in different mixes of such activities as diagnosis and treatment of illness, counseling, provision of day care, and the provision of information and other educational modalities, among many others.

The challenges in designing processes that form part of a program or project's logic model include decisions such as the basic methods through which services will be provided. For example, will services be provided to individual patients/customers? Will services be provided in a congregate setting or even in the homes of patients/customers? Within each service a program or project provides, there is a specific set of tasks that determine how the service is provided. For example, provision of counseling services in a drug-treatment program could involve the following tasks:

- Intake and screening of patients/customers
- Case planning by a counselor
- Implementation of the case plan
- Monitoring of service provision processes by a manager
- Evaluation of the effects of services for the patient/customer
- Termination of the patient/customer from services at completion
- Follow-up of patient/customer's status and progress

Designing the processes component of a program or project's logic model is a complicated undertaking. Adding the design of inputs/resources and the determination of desired results suggests the extent of the challenge in designing a complete logic model as depicted in Figure 1.1. This challenge is further extended by the fact that logic models are not static; they undergo continual revision throughout the life of a program or project.

Even when the initial design of a program or project's logic model is complete, however, managers engage in another major aspect of their designing work.

They also create the *organization design* of their program or project by establishing the intentional patterns of relationships among human and other resources within it.

Creating Organization Designs

Before discussing the specific nature of creating organization designs, it will be useful to provide a brief history of the contemporary concepts that guide designs for programs, projects, and many other types of organizations. For those who prefer contemporary things and ideas, it is sometimes difficult to appreciate old ideas and concepts. It would be a mistake, however, to overlook the historical roots of what is known about organization design.

Although they have been modified over the years, many of the fundamental organization design concepts that guide how most health programs and projects are structured can be traced back to the early twentieth century. The concepts are based on the work of people such as the French industrialist Henri Fayol (1949) and a German sociologist, Max Weber (1947). The work of these and other organization and management theorists of the period, such as Gulick and Urwick (1937) and Mooney and Reiley (1931), resulted in what are now considered the *classical* concepts of organization design.

Perhaps the fact that so many basic design characteristics of contemporary health programs and projects–indeed, of all types of organizations–are rooted in conceptualizations that are nearly a century old reflects the wisdom that went into the development of the classical concepts. Since the classical concepts strongly influence the design of almost all contemporary organizations, including health programs and projects, their role in creating effective contemporary designs must be understood.

Key Concepts in Organization Design

Although many of the classical concepts of organization design remain relevant to the design of modern organizations, including contemporary health programs and projects, the applications of these ideas and concepts have evolved over time. Thus, the following sections present the classical concepts of organization design that are most relevant to health programs and projects. A contemporary perspective on each of the classical concepts is also presented.

Every organized human activity, whether a team playing in a Little League baseball game or the operation of Microsoft Corporation, has two fundamental and opposing requirements: division of the work to be performed on the one hand, and coordination or integration of the divided work on the other. The classical theorists recognized the relationship between dividing work and the concomitant need to coordinate the divided work if satisfactory results are to be achieved. They developed views on division and coordination of work, as well as on other design concepts. In the following section, attention is given to the division of work and the closely associated specialization of workers. Other sections cover authority and responsibility relationships, clustering or departmentalization, span of control, and the coordination or integration of the work that has been consciously divided and performed by specialized workers.

Division of Work and Specialization of Workers

Mintzberg (1983) points out that individual positions in organization designs form the foundation upon which all designs—including entire organizations and systems of organizations—are ultimately constructed. Before Mintzberg and other contemporary thinkers, however, the classical theorists, and even before them the economist Adam Smith (who wrote *The Wealth of Nations* in 1776), recognized the potential inherent in attention to individual positions in organization designs. These theorists recognized the benefits to be gained from dividing work in ways that could maximize the ability of workers occupying individual positions to gain proficiency in their work through specialization.

Technically, division of work means dividing the work to be performed in a program or project (or in any organization) into specific jobs, each consisting of specified activities. The content of a job is determined by the activities a person holding the job is to accomplish. For example, the job of pharmacist in a drug-counseling program is defined by the activities a person in this position is expected to accomplish. These activities are different than those expected of someone with the job of nurse, program manager, or social worker.

Specialists do much of the work in health programs and projects. Their specialized capabilities are often reflected in professional licensure and in accreditation rules and policies that require the programs and projects that hire them to employ people who have met specific licensure and certification requirements (that is, to employ people who are properly *credentialed* for the work they do). Specialization, including but not limited to that which is documented by licensure or certification, implies expertise based on education, experience, or both, in the activities of a job. Health programs and projects are often structured to accommodate the specialties of the participants who work in them through clustering groups of participants according to specialty.

Dividing work and specializing workers enhances managers' ability to select, train, and equip people to do the work of programs and projects. Division of work also permits managers a greater degree of control over work because they can more easily standardize and monitor specialized work and workers. However, increased division of work has a negative side. People who perform highly specialized work may at times find it repetitive, monotonous, and unfulfilling.

In response, such contemporary developments as *cross training* (equipping people with skills that permit them to perform more than one job), *job enlargement* (combining tasks to create a new job involving a broader set of activities), and *job enrichment* (expanding responsibilities so work becomes more challenging and satisfying) permits managers to minimize the negative effects of division and specialization. For example, some health care organizations have established programs that feature integrated patient care teams. Such teams reflect job enrichment efforts that involve each member in team decisions and total care of patients. Cardiac rehabilitation teams, for example, work together to diagnose, treat, rehabilitate, and provide extended care, as a team, from the point of a patient's initial incident through recovery.

Authority and Responsibility Relationships

Growing directly out of the division of work in creating organization designs is the need to assign the responsibility for and authority over the performance of the work. *Authority* is the power derived from a person's structural position in an organization design. Organizational authority permits managers to give orders and to expect that orders be carried out. *Responsibility* is the obligation to perform certain activities or to achieve certain results and, like authority, organizational responsibility is derived from one's position in the organization design.

Authority and responsibility are delegated downward, resulting in a scaling or grading of levels of authority and responsibility. The authority and responsibility of a program or project's manager are different than those of managers of its sub-divisions, as well as those of individual participants. Vertical layers in an organization design are the clearest evidence of the delegation of authority and responsibility. This process of delegation results in what is called a scalar *chain of command* within the organization design. Individuals higher up in the chain have more authority than those lower in the chain. This scalar chain helps define authority and responsibility relationships from the manager down to the level of individual participants.

Classical theorists were obsessed with the role of authority and responsibility in organization designs. In their view, the assignment of authority and responsibility held organizations together. Furthermore, they believed that the rights attached to one's position were the only important sources of power or influence in organizations. The effect of this was to view managers as all-powerful in their organizations. This might have been true 100 years ago, but no longer. Now, authority, especially positional authority, is seen as just one element in the larger concept of interpersonal power in contemporary organization designs.

There are numerous sources of interpersonal power, which has been defined as the ability to influence others in all types of organizational settings, including health programs and projects. The authority that derives from one's formal position is only one source of power. French and Raven (1959) conceptualized interpersonal power as having five distinct bases in organization designs: legitimate, reward, coercive, expert, and referent. Only the first three bases derive from a manager's formal position in a design.

The base of what French and Raven call *legitimate power* is clearly derived from one's position in an organization design. This formal authority resides in managers and exists because organizations find it advantageous to assign power to individuals so they can do their jobs effectively. All managers have some legitimate power or authority based on position. Managers also have *reward power,* which is based on their ability to reward desirable behavior and stems from the legitimate power granted to managers. Because of their positions, managers control rewards such as pay increases, promotions, and work schedules, and this buttresses their legitimate power. Based on their position, managers also have *coercive power,* the opposite of reward power. Coercive power is based on the ability to punish or prevent someone from obtaining desired rewards.

By definition, the legitimate (or positional), reward, and coercive sources of power in organization designs are restricted to managers. However, other sources of power not restricted to managers exist in organization design. These other sources are quite important in health programs and projects and have the effect of spreading power and influence beyond the managers.

One of the most important forms of power in many programs and projects is *expert power,* which is derived from having knowledge that is valued within the program or project, or by an organization in which it is embedded. Expert power is personal to the person who has the expertise. Thus, it is different from legitimate, reward, and coercive power, which are prescribed by the organization design, even though persons may be granted these types of power because they possess expert power. For example, health professionals with expert power often rise to management positions in their areas of expertise. In addition, in programs or projects where work is highly technical or professional, expert power alone can make certain people powerful. In any program or project, participants with scarce expertise will typically have more expert power than people whose expertise is more readily replicable.

What French and Raven call *referent power* results when someone engenders admiration, loyalty, and emulation to the extent that the person gains the power to influence other people. Sometimes called charismatic power, this form of power is certainly not limited to managers. In some health programs and projects, charismatic individuals wield considerable influence. As with expert power, referent power cannot be given by the organization, although legitimate, reward, and coercive power can be.

Authority and responsibility considerations heavily influence the design of contemporary organizations, including health programs and projects. However, the contemporary view expands on the classical concept and views positional authority as only one of several sources of power. In this larger perspective, power is not limited to managers. A broader discussion of power and influence can be found in Chapter Four.

Clustering

The process of clustering or grouping work and workers into manageable units (see Figure 3.1) heavily influences organization designs. The classical view of clustering—or as the classicists preferred to call it, departmentalization—is that it is a natural consequence of division and specialization of work. In their view, because it is rational to specialize work, it is also rational to place similar workers together in work groups. In turn, these groups are grouped into clusters of related work groups until the organization design has a superstructure.

Gulick and Urwick (1937), among other classicists, noted four bases for clustering work and workers: purpose, process, persons and things, and place. Other factors upon which clustering can be based have emerged. Mintzberg (1979), for example, suggests six bases for grouping workers into units and units into larger units. Workers can be grouped on the basis of the following:

Specialized knowledge and skills	A health program might group nurses in one unit and social workers in another.
Functions or processes performed	A large program might have marketing, finance, and clinical services units.
Timing of their work	A program that operates twenty-four hours per day might group workers into day, evening, and night shifts.
Outputs of their work, whether by services or products	A program might group workers by whether they provide inpatient or outpatient services.

Clients or patients they serve

Programs might be established based on age or gender of patients, such as geriatric or women's health programs.

Place or physical location of their work

A program might operate ambulatory clinics in a downtown location as well as in the city's suburbs.

A single large health program or project might use several of these bases for grouping workers in order to create an effective organization design. Larger organizations in which programs and projects are housed use many, if not all, of these bases for clustering to create their designs.

No matter which basis is used, the clustering of work and workers into manageable units helps establish the means by which their work can be integrated and coordinated, both within the groups and with other work groups. Mintzberg (1979) suggests that clustering has at least four important implications for participants and the organization designs within which they work:

- Clustering sets up a system of common supervision. Once participants are clustered, a manager can be appointed to integrate and control the work of the group.
- Clustering facilitates sharing resources. People in work groups share a common budget, facilities, and equipment.
- Clustering typically leads to common measures of performance. Shared resources on the input side and group-level outputs and outcomes permit group members to be evaluated by common performance criteria. (Recall the earlier discussion about appraising teams in this chapter.) Common performance measures encourage group members to integrate their work.
- Clustering encourages communication. Shared inputs/resources and shared desired outputs, outcomes, and impact, along with close physical proximity, encourages communication. This facilitates integrating the work of group members.

Health programs and projects, as well as larger organizations in which they might be embedded, use all six of the bases discussed previously for clustering work and participants, including doing so by function, the basis most favored by the classical theorists. This basis, reinforced by the specialized knowledge and skills of many participants in health programs and projects, is clearly visible in large health programs where nurses are in one cluster, pharmacists are in another, and social workers are in yet another cluster. In smaller programs or projects, this functional basis is less frequently used and clustering is more likely to be based on patients/customers served or on physical location.

One important contemporary development in the organization designs of many health programs and projects—as well as the organizations in which they may be embedded—is the increased focus on patients/customers as the basis for clustering participants. This is one result of the increased competition for patients/ customers. For example, as the leaders of health care organizations seek to devise business strategies to increase the market shares their organizations hold, many have initiated geriatric and women's health programs and comprehensive cardiac care programs marketed specifically to corporate executives.

Clustering Participants into Work Groups or Teams. As Figure 3.1 indicates, the first level of clustering in organization designs is the grouping of individual participants into work groups or teams. Projects and smaller programs are typically organized as teams. Frequently, the participants form a single team; it may even be called the project team. Larger programs may contain a number of teams.

Groups and teams are established within organization designs for many purposes. For example, large organizations establish management teams, governing boards, and standing committees. Some groups are assembled for specific problem-solving purposes or to pursue improvements in quality or productivity. Problem-solving and improvement-oriented teams are ubiquitous in health services settings. More is said about teams and teamwork in Chapter Nine, where the role of teamwork in continuous improvement is discussed. The focus here, however, is on the formal work of teams made up of the participants in programs and projects.

Because the work team is vital to the success of a program or project, managers should view one of their important responsibilities as *team building* or *team development* (Beyerlein, Johnson, and Beyerlein 2000). Team building or development includes enhancing the ability of individual participants to contribute to team performance by providing education and training, by increasing their motivation to perform as individuals and team members, and by enhancing the capability of the team to perform as a team.

An important aspect of building and developing work teams is the realization that all teams, including work teams, form in a series of evolving stages (Tuckman and Jensen 1977; Fried, Topping, and Rundall 2000; Ashmos 1998; McConnell 2003). Although not all teams evolve in precisely the same manner, typically the evolution of a work team involves several discernable stages, beginning with a *formation* stage that occurs when a team is first established. Team participants in this stage sort out their roles and those of other participants as they begin to identify themselves as part of a team and to try to determine what is acceptable within the group.

Formation is followed by a stage variously characterized as *storming, disequilibrium,* or *differentiation.* This stage is characterized by real and potential conflicts among team participants. Managers can play important roles in moving teams beyond this stage by building trust and respect among participants and by clarifying roles of individuals and of the entire team. Some teams never emerge from this stage, and this stage as its name suggests is always "stormy."

For teams that do progress, the next stage is characterized as the *norming, integrating,* or *achieving role clarity* stage. Agreement is reached regarding roles, and cohesion among team participants increases significantly. Team members begin to identify with the desired results established for the team and the program or project within which the team works, and to develop or reaffirm shared values. Communication flows relatively easily within the team as participants gain trust and familiarity with each other.

Successful teams evolve further to a *maturity* stage or what is sometimes called the *performing* stage. In this stage, the organization design for team participants is well-established, and participants are concerned about the team and its effectiveness. Teams at this stage are able to effectively accomplish the team's work and to deal with conflicts within the team. Participants are aware of one another's strengths and weaknesses and accept their differences. Typically, participants in teams at the mature stage experience satisfaction with their work, enjoy high levels of cooperation, mutual trust, and support among team members, and experience pride in the accomplishments of the team.

Importantly, a team's maturity is not an endpoint. A team's effectiveness—including both work accomplishment and participant satisfaction—must be maintained, which can be thought of as a new stage. Perhaps more accurately, this is not so much a new stage as a continuation of the performing stage, accomplished through significant and ongoing efforts to maintain the team's effectiveness.

For some health programs and projects, a work team's final evolutionary stage is reached when the team dissolves or adjourns. Most health projects have a finite life span that is determined at the outset. For them, this final stage is a natural conclusion of the project. On the other hand, plans for programs typically include an indefinite life span. The *adjournment* or *dissolution* stage for programs and for projects before their planned termination date may result from changes in the strategies of the organizations in which they are embedded, perhaps driven by changes in the markets for services, or from changes in reimbursement policy. Dissolution may also result from a program or project's failure to achieve its desired results. Some programs and projects simply fail and are terminated.

Span of Control

A fundamental organization design question of concern to the classical theorists was how large clusters of workers could be and still be effective. A related question was how to make decisions about the size of clusters. In considering these questions classical theorists developed the organization design concept called *span of control,* which is defined as the number of organizational subordinates reporting directly to an organizational superior. Classical theorists generally agreed that managers should have a limited number of people reporting directly to them. Their conclusion was based on their view of the ability of managers to exercise the necessary degree of control over those whom they managed.

Spans of control significantly affect organization designs. As seen in Figure 3.3, narrow spans of control produce *tall* organization designs, and wider spans produce *flat* organization designs. The tall and flat structures in Figure 3.3 have equal numbers of positions, but the tall structure has four levels, while the flat one has two. Complex health organizations (such as hospitals or large health departments) typically have tall patterns resulting from extensive division of work and concurrent specialization of workers into numerous and varied departments and units. This tall pattern results from the need to have limited spans of control when work is highly divided and performed by specialized workers. In contrast, health programs and projects typically have flat designs.

FIGURE 3.3. CONTRASTING SPANS OF CONTROL.

A Tall Complex Organization

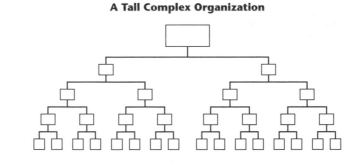

A Flat Health Program or Project

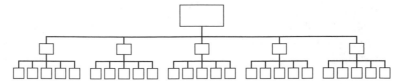

The factors contemporary managers use to determine an appropriate span of control include the following:

Level of professionalism and training of participants	Professional, highly trained participants (characteristics often prevalent among participants in health programs and projects) require less supervision, which permits wider spans of control.
Level of uncertainty in the work being done	Complex and varied work requires close supervision when compared to simple and repetitive work. Close supervision requires narrow spans of control.
Degree of standardization of work	Standardized and routinized work requires less direct supervision. Spans of control for standardized work can be wider than for less standardized work.
Degree of interaction required between managers and other participants	Work situations in which more interaction is needed between managers and other participants require narrower spans of control because effective interactions take time.
Degree of task integration required	If the work being done by participants must be carefully coordinated or integrated, or if the various aspects of work are interdependent, a narrower span of control may be needed.

The classical concept of span of control remains highly relevant to the design of health programs and projects, although several contingencies must be considered when applying the concept. The manager of a large program with four or five separate units may find that the heads of these units constitute an appropriate span of control. At levels of the program where work is standardized and routine the spans could be much wider.

Another determining factor in span of control decisions is the nature of the work. It is usually easier to supervise ten data processors than five drug counselors. Also, the abilities and availability of managers must be taken into account. The training and personal qualities of some managers enable them to manage broader spans of control than others can manage. Similarly, better training and higher potential for self-direction of those being managed reduces the need for relationships with their managers and widens the spans the managers can handle.

Coordination or Integration

Coordination and *integration* are used interchangeably in the organization design literature. Whichever term is used, the concept pertains to processes intended to achieve unity of effort among the various component parts in an organization design in the accomplishment of its desired results. Although the focus here is on integration within programs and projects, the concept applies to the entire hierarchy of organization designs shown in Figure 3.1.

As was noted previously, health programs and projects can exhibit high degrees of division of work and specialization of workers. When they do, there is a greater need for effective coordination. While in some situations it is possible to separate work so as to minimize the degree of coordination needed, health programs and projects typically require much coordination if their missions and objectives are to be achieved. It is important to recognize the interaction between the need to divide, specialize, and cluster work and participants, and subsequent requirements for coordination. More differentiation of work and specialization of participants increases the need for coordination.

The value of effective coordination is also influenced by the type of interdependence existing among participants in a program or project. Thompson (1967) identifies three forms of interdependence, pooled, sequential, and reciprocal. All three are found in health programs and projects. *Pooled interdependence* occurs when individual participants or work groups are related, but not closely. They simply contribute separately in some way to the larger whole. For example, several geographically dispersed units of a drug-counseling program housed in a single health department can be viewed as linked largely in the sense that each contributes to the overall success of the program; however, they have very little direct interdependence. They operate as separate entities for all practical purposes.

Sequential interdependence occurs when individual participants or work groups bear a close and sequential connection. For example, patients/customers enrolled in a large multi-service program become the focal point for extended chains of sequentially interdependent activities. The program's intake office enrolls them and schedules an initial evaluation of their status and needs. This may trigger separate appointments with a nurse, social worker, and physical therapist, all occurring in a sequentially interdependent manner.

The third type of interdependence, *reciprocal interdependence,* occurs when individual participants or work groups bear a close relationship and the interdependence moves in both directions. For example, a hospice program might exist to serve patients of a particular health care organization or system. The hospice relies upon the organization as its source of patients, and the organization relies upon the hospice as a place to refer appropriate patients. The interdependence is reciprocal because it moves in both directions.

Typically, as interdependence moves from pooled, to sequential, to reciprocal, managers must pay greater attention to issues of coordination. Health programs and projects typically exhibit very high levels of internal interdependence among their component parts, usually of the sequential or reciprocal forms. Some also have high levels of interdependence with the organizations in which they are embedded. Thus, the need for effective coordination is usually significant in health programs and projects.

Mechanisms for Achieving Coordination. The mechanisms of coordination—the techniques and processes managers use to achieve coordination—are diverse and result in different levels of success depending upon characteristics of specific situations. No single coordinating mechanism is best for all situations. Managers need to match the most appropriate coordinating mechanism to a given situation, recognizing that often a combination of mechanisms is required.

Managers can select from a large menu of mechanisms of coordination, typically choosing and applying several of them simultaneously. A number of categorizations of these mechanisms have been developed. One categorization (Litterer 1965) outlines the following three ways for managers to achieve coordination:

- Using an organization design's hierarchical structure
- Relying upon administrative systems and procedures such as reporting mechanisms
- Relying upon participants to voluntarily coordinate their work as needed

Hierarchical coordination relies upon having the various participants in a program or project placed under a single line of managerial authority. In small and relatively simple organization designs typical of many programs and projects, this form of coordination is very effective. However, in large complex programs and projects, and in other larger organization designs with multiple organizational levels and many sub-divisions, hierarchical coordination becomes more difficult as a means of achieving coordination.

Although a program or project's manager is a focal point of authority, it may be impossible for one person to cope with all the coordinating problems that might arise in the hierarchy. Therefore, coordination through the hierarchical structure is almost always supplemented by other mechanisms.

A second mechanism suggested by Litterer is the incorporation of *formal procedures and administrative systems* into a program or project's organization design. Such procedures and systems can be as simple as routing certain information to the set of participants whose work is to be coordinated. To the extent that administrative procedures can be programmed or made routine, they are easy to use. For non-routine and non-programmable events, other administrative procedures, such as establishing committees, may also provide coordination within a program or project.

A third type of coordination mechanism in Litterer's view is the *voluntary actions of participants* undertaken to ensure coordination in a program or project. In many health programs and projects, much of the coordination does in fact depend upon the willingness and ability of participants to voluntarily find ways to integrate or coordinate their activities with other participants.

Managers can facilitate voluntary coordination by providing participants with a good knowledge of the program or project's logic model and with information concerning specific problems of coordination. If this can be coupled with the motivation to do something about coordination problems, voluntary coordination routinely occurs. In part, such motivation stems from the professionalism of so many of the participants in health programs and projects. Their value systems, which are supportive of patients/customers' welfare, facilitate voluntary coordination.

In a second important categorization of mechanisms of coordination available to managers, Mintzberg (1983) identifies the following five mechanisms:

- Mutual adjustment
- Direct supervision
- Standardization of work processes
- Standardization of work outputs
- Standardization of worker skills

In *mutual adjustment,* which is quite similar to the voluntary actions identified by Litterer, coordination is achieved through the willingness of participants to coordinate work through mutual adjustments to each other's needs. Managers facilitate this mechanism by encouraging communication among those whose work must be coordinated. This mechanism to achieve coordination is especially useful in self-directed work teams.

In *direct supervision,* which is similar to the hierarchical coordination identified by Litterer, coordination is achieved by having certain participants take responsibility for the work of others, including issuing instructions to them and monitoring their actions. This occurs as a matter of course in the relationship between managers and those they manage.

In *standardization of work processes,* the content of work is programmed or specified in advance. Health programs and projects routinely standardize many of their work processes such as intake procedures for patients/customers. They also standardize work processes through the establishment of patient care protocols or clinical pathways for guiding the provision of services.

The *standardization of outputs* as a coordinating mechanism involves the specification of the product or output of work, with determination of how to perform the work left to the worker. Professional work is often more readily coordinated through mechanisms that standardize outputs than through attempts to standardize the work processes.

Finally, when neither work processes nor outputs can be standardized, Mintzberg suggests that coordination can be achieved through *standardization of worker skills,* which is accomplished through training, education, and experience. This coordination mechanism is frequently used in health programs and projects in which the complexity of much of the work does not allow standardization of work processes or outputs. In such situations, standardization of participant skills and knowledge can be an excellent coordinating mechanism. It is routine for teams of physicians, nurses, and other clinicians to coordinate their care of patients largely through this mechanism. It also helps explain why membership on such teams is highly interchangeable.

Hage (1980) offers a third useful categorization of coordinating mechanisms in which he suggests the following four mechanisms:

- Programming (developing rules and prescriptions for how to do things)
- Planning
- Customs
- Feedback

In Hage's view, managers use *programming* to accomplish coordination by specifying what work is to be done in each individual position in a program or project, as well as how it is to be done. They can also specify the relationships among clusters of individual positions, up to the level of entire organizations and systems. With such guidance, participants can learn their jobs and conduct their work in a coordinated manner. The programming in an organization design is accomplished through rules, manuals, job descriptions, personnel procedures, promotion policies, and so on. This type of coordinating mechanism is quite similar to Litterer's use of administrative systems and procedures, and to Mintzberg's standardization of work, processes, and skills. These mechanisms of coordination are pervasive in many health programs and projects.

The usefulness of *planning* as a coordination mechanism is obvious when viewing plans for one part of a program or project in relationship to plans for other parts of the program or project, or when viewing plans for an entire program or project in relationship to plans for its organizational home. For example, the plans of a program or project must take into account the expansion plans of its organizational home. Similarly, subunit plans within a large program or project must take into account the plans of the entire program or project. Coordination is facilitated when managers make sure their plans are compatible with all other relevant plans.

Customs are a frequently overlooked coordination mechanism. Yet, many managers rely heavily upon the history and customs of their programs or projects, or the organizations in which they are embedded, as coordination mechanisms. For example, it may be customary in a particular long-term care organization to use the holiday season as an occasion to invite the families of residents into the facility for a meal and social interaction. Advanced knowledge of this custom permits the various departments, programs, and projects to begin preparing for this event well in advance and facilitates the coordination of their various contributions to its success. Customs alone, however, are rarely sufficient to fully meet the coordination challenge.

The final mechanism in Hage's categorization, *feedback,* may indicate when a program or project, or some component of it, is not functioning well; feedback can trigger renewed efforts to coordinate work. Feedback often takes the form of written reports on operations and activities in health programs or projects, but it also includes the verbal exchanges that occur between and among participants. All forms of effective communication include feedback, as discussed in Chapter Six.

Feedback often occurs in the context of *committees* or *teams,* which actually form another coordination mechanism. Some of these groups are made up of participants from subunits of a large program or project for the specific purpose of achieving coordination among the subunits. Using committees or teams for purposes of coordination is a well-established approach in health programs and projects. Of course, committees and teams serve other purposes besides coordination, including performing service, and filling advisory or decision-making roles.

Selecting from the Menu of Coordinating Mechanisms. In order to achieve coordination within their programs and projects, managers have available a rich menu of mechanisms, as was discussed in the previous sections. Managers can select from a menu that includes the following:

- Administrative systems and procedures
- Committees and teams
- Customs
- Direct supervision
- Feedback

- Hierarchy
- Mutual adjustment
- Planning
- Programming
- Standardization of work processes, outputs, or worker skills
- Voluntary action

Managers typically use various combinations of these mechanisms to achieve coordination, often using several of them concurrently.

Depending upon the circumstances, use of various packages or sets of these mechanisms can be tailored appropriately. For example, a manager concerned about how a program or project is coordinated with other parts of the organization in which it is embedded, might select a particular set of coordination mechanisms. The managers of the subunits of this program or project, concerned about coordination among the subunits, would choose a different package of mechanisms. The manager of one of the units, a pharmacy for example, concerned about coordination issues involved in the proper dispensing of pharmaceuticals, might select yet another set of mechanisms.

Application of the Key Organization Design Concepts

The influence of the design concepts examined previously (for example, division of work and specialization of participants, authority and responsibility relationships, clustering, span of control, and coordination) on the actual organization designs of contemporary health programs and projects—as well as on the larger organizations in which they are often embedded—is readily seen in the schematic representation of an organization design known as an *organization chart*. For example, the simplified organization chart in Figure 3.4 reflects the consequences of applying the organization design concepts to a large health organization. The result is the classic functional organization design so ubiquitous in business, government, academia, and health care.

Each unit in the chart represents a *division of work* and suggests that participants in each unit do work for which they are *specialized*. The chart also has lines representing *authority and responsibility relationships* between organizational superiors and subordinates. The vertical dimension of the organization chart shows who has authority over and responsibility for who and what. Participants who are higher in the chart generally have authority over those in lower positions. Participants on the same level generally have equal amounts of authority and responsibility.

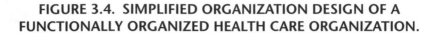

FIGURE 3.4. SIMPLIFIED ORGANIZATION DESIGN OF A FUNCTIONALLY ORGANIZED HEALTH CARE ORGANIZATION.

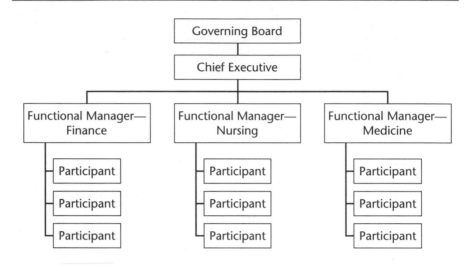

The chart also depicts *clustering* of individual participants into units, with the process being based primarily on functions (for example finance, nursing, medicine). The chart permits an assessment of the *span of control* at various points simply by counting the participants reporting to any manager. Finally, because multiple interdependent or interrelated units are depicted, the importance of *coordinating* work can be seen in this organization chart. However, the chart does not suggest what mechanisms might be used to achieve coordination.

Figure 3.5 illustrates that the organization design of a program or project can also be a classical functionally designed structure. The program or project illustrated in this figure could be freestanding and independent, in which case it might have a governing body of its own. It could be the result of a joint venture between two organizations, in which case it might report to both of them. Most typically, however, it would be embedded in a larger functionally organized organization as shown in Figure 3.6.

There are organization designs in which almost all work is done through programs or projects. Many architectural, engineering, and consulting firms are organized into projects and derive their revenues from performing these projects for clients. Other organizations, including certain construction firms, defense contractors, and other government contractors, are organized by programs. Figure 3.7 illustrates the extreme form of what might be called a "programmized" or "projectized" organization.

FIGURE 3.5. SIMPLIFIED ORGANIZATION DESIGN OF A FUNCTIONALLY ORGANIZED PROGRAM OR PROJECT.

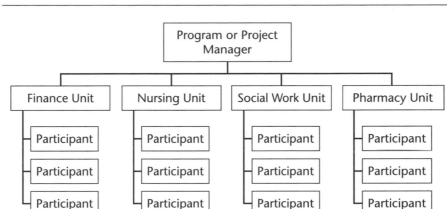

The *matrix* organization design shown in Figure 3.8 blends elements of the classic functional design depicted in Figure 3.4 and the "programmized" or "projectized" design shown in Figure 3.7. This organization design is widely used for health programs and projects embedded in larger organizations.

To illustrate an example of a matrix design, consider how a health care organization might design a comprehensive home health program for the chronically ill. This would require a work group organized around the focus of the program (home services for the chronically ill). Participants in the group could be drawn from a variety of functional units of the organization, including nursing, social services, respiratory therapy, occupational therapy, pharmacy, and physicians specializing in chronic disease. To market the program and to handle finance and reimbursement issues, participants with such expertise could be drawn from these areas of the organization in which the program is embedded. A program manager would be named and given authority over and overall responsibility for the program. The manager would report to a superior in the larger organization in which the program is housed.

Health care organizations create matrix organization designs when they superimpose programs or projects on their existing functionally clustered designs. The programs and projects do not replace the functionally organized design; they are organic complements to the more mechanistic functional structure and eliminate some of its rigidity in certain circumstances. Matrix designs are especially useful for projects that tend to have a limited scope and finite life, projects to design and implement an electronic medical record or to design an offsite clinic for example.

FIGURE 3.6. ORGANIZATION DESIGN WITH PROGRAM OR PROJECT EMBEDDED IN A HEALTH CARE ORGANIZATION

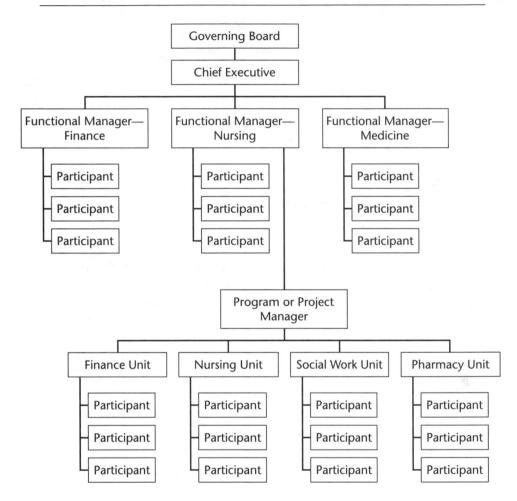

Contemporary health care organizations contain a variety of organization designs. In most of them, their structures feature classic functionally organized designs. Some of the programs and projects embedded within them may also have classic functional designs. Others may use matrix designs. As was noted earlier in this chapter, however, no matter how managers build the formal organization designs of their programs and projects, coexisting within the formal organization design will be an informal structure.

FIGURE 3.7. "PROGRAMMIZED" OR "PROJECTIZED" ORGANIZATION DESIGN.

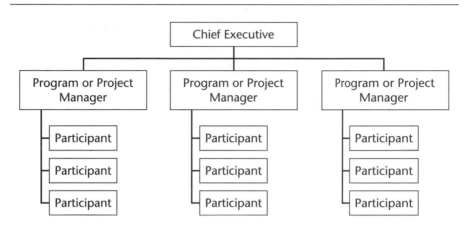

FIGURE 3.8. MATRIX ORGANIZATION DESIGN.

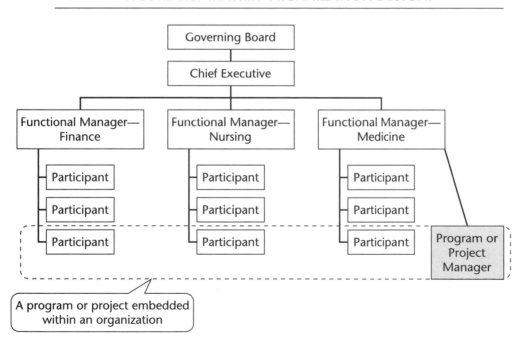

Managers neither establish nor fully control the informal aspects of organization designs. Instead, the other participants, according to their preferences and wishes, establish informal relationships and activities within the formal designs because people working together invariably establish relationships and interactions outside the formal structure. Thus, it is important for program and project managers to understand both the formal and the informal aspects of organization designs.

Informal Aspects of Organization Designs

The informal relationships that occur within formal organization designs are characterized by dynamic behavior and patterns that occur as a result of people working with other people across formal design parameters. Informal relationships are established as people in organizational settings interact to accomplish work within the context of the formal organization design, as well as for other more personal reasons such as a desire for friendships and social interaction.

Figure 3.9 illustrates some of the actual contacts that might occur between participants in an organization design. As can be seen, not all contacts follow the formal paths. In some of the contacts, levels of the organization are bypassed; in others there is cross contact from one chain of command in the organization to another. While contact charts do not show the reasons for informal relationships, they do reflect the nature of the informal relationships that can arise within organization designs.

Informal Groups within Organization Designs

In addition to the one-to-one informal relationships shown in Figure 3.9, fully drawn contact charts often show a type of clustering that occurs outside the formal organization design. Groups within organization designs can be either formally or informally established. As was discussed previously in the section on clustering, managers intentionally cluster participants into formal groups such as committees or teams as a means of achieving certain purposes. In contrast, informal groups arise from the propensity of people to form *social* groups.

People seek to fulfill a variety of their needs through work and within the context in which the work is performed. If formal organization designs satisfied all the needs of participants there would be no reason to establish or engage in informal relationships. Basically, informal interactions occur because participants' needs are not fully met by the formal organization design. In fact, many needs can best be met in the context of informal relationships and groups.

FIGURE 3.9. A CONTACT CHART.

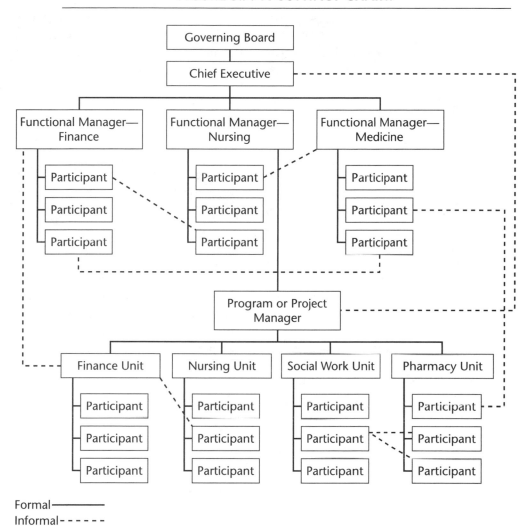

Formal————
Informal------

Interpersonal contacts within small informal groups provide relief from the boredom, monotony, and pressures of the workplace. In groups, people can be with others with similar values and interests. Groups may accord their members status, which may be little more than a sense of belonging to a group that is more or less exclusive. Informal group membership also provides a degree of personal security; the group member feels acceptance by peers as an equal and feels secure in their company. Group membership permits the individual to express views to sympathetic listeners. Group members may even find outlets for leadership drives. Finally, group membership assists people in securing information, at least information of a certain type. The grapevine–the flow of communication through informal channels as described in Chapter Six–is a phenomenon known to all participants in organization designs. The common denominator in all these reasons for group membership is the satisfaction of specific needs of members that are not fully met by the formal organization. It is very important for managers to understand that informal groups arise and persist within organization designs because they perform desired functions for their members.

The Structure of Informal Groups. Informal groups that form within organization designs tend to develop complex structures of relationships of their own. These structures are determined by different status positions of a group's members: group leader, primary group member, fringe group member, and out status. For example, Figure 3.10 shows the informal structure of a group of nine people working in one section of a large health program. The solid square in the center includes the group leader. Clustered around the leader are the other four members of the primary group. This close association is characterized by intense interaction and communication. The three people at the fringe are likely to be newcomers who are, in effect, being evaluated by the primary group and who may become full members. If not accepted, however, they will move to out

FIGURE 3.10. INFORMAL GROUP STRUCTURE.

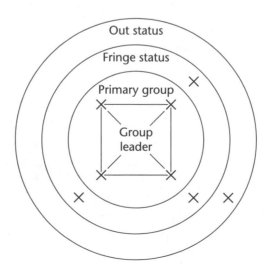

status. One person is already in out status. This has significant implications if the person in out status wants to belong to the primary group. Being a participant in the formal organization design of this program is no substitute for full membership in the informal group.

An important parameter of how informal groups function is their leadership, even if it is unofficial or unsanctioned within the formal organization design. Informal group leaders emerge from within groups because they serve several functions. The leader not only initiates action and provides direction, but also resolves differences of opinion on group-related matters and conflicts between or among the group's members. Furthermore, the leader can communicate group values and feelings to representatives of the formal organization design. The informal group leadership role is retained only as long as the role is performed well; a group's members grant the leadership role and they can take it away.

Managers' Responses to Informal Relationships within Organization Designs

Because the informal relationships within organization designs are not established by managers, nor are they as controllable by them as are the various formal aspects of a design, managers sometimes view informal relationships as problems. These relationships can indeed be problematic, but they can also serve useful purposes for managers. They can be blended with the formal organization design of a program or project to help facilitate the accomplishment of its mission and objectives with quality and efficiency.

Sometimes formal organization designs are too inflexible to meet the needs of a dynamic situation. Thus, the more flexible and spontaneous characteristics of informal relationships—such as the speed of communication through the grapevine—can have advantages. In emergencies, for example, the informal relationships and arrangements existing within a formal design may preserve the organization from the harm that could result from strict adherence to formal channels of communication or literal obedience to the rules and regulations governing who does what.

Another potential advantage of informal relationships is that when informal group support is available to the manager, management work is easier. Managers can delegate and decentralize authority and responsibility more easily when informal groups are cooperative. The converse of this is also true; in the absence of informal group support, management work is more difficult. To protect themselves and to make their work situation acceptable, people typically resist what they perceive as autocratic management. The resistance often takes place within the context of informal relationships and arrangements and may take the form of such undesirable outcomes as work restriction, insubordination, or disloyalty.

The performance level achieved by any program or project is affected by its participants' willingness to grant cooperation and enthusiasm. Managers who understand this and who understand that the co-existence of the formal and informal aspects of organization designs is a fact of life will take steps to balance the formal and informal aspects. A suitable balance may be difficult to achieve, but managers can do two things to move toward this balance.

First, they can seek to understand the informal relationships and arrangements that exist among the participants in their programs and projects, and demonstrate their understanding and acceptance of them. Particularly important in conveying acceptance is for managers to minimize the negative effect of their actions on the often-fragile informal relationships and arrangements. Above all, managers should realize that attempting to suppress informal relationships and arrangements creates destructive and dysfunctional situations.

Second, managers can work to integrate the interests of the formal and informal aspects of their organization designs. In so doing they should avoid formal organization design features that unnecessarily threaten or diminish the quality of informal relationships and arrangements. In effect, blending the informal relationships and arrangements that exist within organization designs with their formal design elements helps establish the organizational culture of the program or project.

The informal relationships among participants in programs and projects are important to the participants, and to the programs and projects as well. The informal aspects of organization design deserve the attention of managers because they can complement the effectiveness of the formal design.

Summary

In designing for effectiveness, managers create logic models and organization designs for their programs and projects. The organization designs of contemporary health programs and projects are created through application of a set of organization design concepts whose roots can be traced back to general administrative theorists who lived early in the twentieth century. Their work established what are called the classical concepts of organization design.

The chapter also includes a discussion of the important dimensions of the informal relationships that people establish within the formal organization designs in which they work, and how managers can tap into the potential for informal features of their designs to contribute to effectiveness.

The classical concept of division of work—dividing the work of a program or project into specific jobs having specified activities—is discussed. For example, the job of pharmacist is defined by the activities a person in this position is expected to accomplish. The corollary of division of work, the specialization of the participants who perform the work, is also discussed.

Growing directly out of the division of work is a need to assign responsibility for and authority over performance of work. This assignment occurs through the technical process of delegation, which results in scaling or grading the levels of authority and responsibility in an organization design.

A natural consequence of division and specialization of work is clustering or grouping (called departmentalization by the classicists) of jobs under the authority of one manager. Six bases for clustering workers are examined: knowledge and skills, work process and function, time, output, client, and place. The span of control concept is examined, with emphasis on the influence of span on the shape (tall or flat) of the organization design. A number of contingency factors that help determine the proper span of control are discussed.

Coordination is described as the process intended to achieve unity of effort among the various parts of an organization design in the accomplishment of its mission and objectives. An extensive menu of coordinating mechanisms available to managers is presented, including the following:

- Administrative systems and procedures
- Committees
- Customs
- Direct supervision
- Feedback
- Hierarchy
- Mutual adjustment
- Planning
- Programming
- Standardization of work processes, outputs, or worker skills
- Voluntary action

The formal and informal aspects of organization design are applied to illustrate a functionally designed organization (Figure 3.4). Figure 3.8 illustrates a matrix organization design, a popular approach to embedding programs and projects in larger organizations.

Chapter Review Questions

1. Discuss the design of logic models for programs and projects.
2. Distinguish between the formal and informal aspects of organization design.
3. Discuss the advantages and disadvantages of dividing work. What are the implications for managers of dividing work?
4. What is the relationship between authority and responsibility in organization designs? Discuss the sources of each.
5. Describe the important bases for clustering in the design of health programs and projects and give an example using each base.
6. What factors should be considered in determining an appropriate span of control within a program or project?
7. Discuss the menu of mechanisms available to managers as they seek to achieve coordination within programs and projects.
8. Why do people form informal groups within formal organization designs?
9. What should managers do about informal groups in their programs or projects?
10. Model and describe the basic staffing process and discuss the interdependence among the steps in the process.

CHAPTER FOUR

LEADING TO ACCOMPLISH DESIRED RESULTS

Managers engage in three highly interrelated core activities as they perform management work: *strategizing, designing,* and *leading* (see Figure 1.3). Strategizing and designing activities are discussed in Chapters Two and Three. This chapter discusses the third core activity of management work, *leading.* It has been established through extensive research that there are positive associations between how well managers perform their leading activities and "follower attitudes, such as trust, job satisfaction, and organizational commitment, and behaviors, such as job performance at the individual, group, and organizational levels" (Bono and Judge 2003, p. 554).

Adapting well-known definitions (Pointer and Sanchez 2000; Yukl 2002), we define leading by managers in programs and projects as influencing others to understand and agree about what needs to be done in order to achieve the desired results established for a program or project and facilitating the individual and collective contributions of others to achievement of the desired results. *Influencing* is the most critical element of the leading activity, "its center of gravity" (Pointer and Sanchez 2000, p. 109). Influence is important to success in leading because it is the means by which "people successfully persuade others to follow their advice, suggestion, or order" (Keys and Case 1990, p. 38).

As will be discussed in this chapter, what managers do when leading is complex and multidimensional, although its essence is one person influencing other people. In his seminal study of leadership, for which he won a Pulitzer Prize,

James Burns identifies the central function of leadership: to achieve a collective purpose (Burns 1978). The focus of this chapter includes ways in which managers can influence and facilitate the contributions of other participants to accomplishing the desired results established for programs and projects. A key aspect of the ability of managers to influence participants' contributions is through the ability of managers to affect the *motivation* of participants to contribute. Thus, attention is also given to motivation. After reading the chapter, the reader should be able to do the following:

- Define leading and understand the relationships between influence and leading and between interpersonal power and influence
- Define motivation and model the motivation process
- Distinguish between the content and process perspectives on motivation and understand the implications of both perspectives for leading
- Understand the main approaches to studies of leading, which include leader traits, leader behaviors, and situational or contingency approaches

Motivation at Work

To be effective at leading the participants involved in a program or project, whether paid staff or volunteers, managers must help create and maintain conditions under which the participants can and do contribute to accomplishing the desired results established for the program or project. Managers must influence other participants to behave in contributory ways. Knowledge of how motivation occurs is a means of understanding why people behave in particular ways. Thus, an understanding of human motivation is necessary for success in leading.

Managers need participants to exhibit a diverse set of contributory behaviors in order for their programs and projects to be successful. At the most basic level, they want participants to join the program or project and attend work regularly, punctually, and predictably. These behaviors do not happen by chance; they are motivated behaviors. Managers also want participants to perform the direct or support work assigned to them in the program or project's logic model and organization design. They want this work to be performed at acceptable levels of quantity and quality. Finally, managers want participants to exhibit good citizenship behaviors, including such specific behaviors as cooperation, altruism, protecting fellow workers and property, and generally going above and beyond the call of duty. The presence of high levels of good citizenship behaviors among the participants in a program or project invariably contributes directly to attaining desired results in the form of outputs, outcomes, and impact. How can managers create and maintain the conditions that cause such desirable behaviors in the participants in their programs and projects? Part of the answer lies in motivating participants to practice the desirable behaviors. Thus, an understanding of motivation in workplaces is crucial to effective leading.

The concept of motivation is at once simple and complex. Motivation is simple because human behavior is goal-directed and is induced by increasingly well-understood forces, some of which are internal to the individual and some of which are external. Motivation is complex because mechanisms that induce behavior include very complicated and individualized needs, wants, and desires that are shaped, affected, and satisfied in different ways for different people. Before exploring the key theories and models that have been developed to explain human motivation in the workplace, it is first necessary to define motivation and model the basic motivation process.

Motivation Defined and Modeled

Why does one participant in a program or project work harder than another? Why is one more cooperative than another? One answer is that people have various needs and behave differently in attempting to fulfill their needs. The needs are, in effect, deficiencies that cause people to undertake patterns of behavior intended to fill the deficiencies. For example, at a very simple level, human needs are physiological. A hungry person needs food, is driven by hunger, and is motivated to satisfy the need for food (in other words, to overcome the deficiency). Other needs are more complex. Some needs are psychological (for example, the need for self-esteem); others are sociological (for example, the need for social interaction). In short, needs in human beings trigger and energize behaviors intended to satisfy the needs. This fact is the basis for a model of how motivation occurs.

As shown in Figure 4.1, the motivation process is cyclical. It begins with an unmet need and cycles through the individual's assessment of the results of efforts to satisfy the need. This assessment may confirm the continuation of an unmet need or permit the identification of a new need. In between, the person searches for ways to satisfy the need, chooses a course of action, and exhibits goal-directed behavior intended to satisfy the unmet need. The model is over-simplified but contains the following essential elements of the process by which human motivation occurs:

- Motivation is driven by unsatisfied or unmet needs.
- Motivation results in goal-directed behaviors to satisfy the unmet needs.
- Motivation can be influenced by factors that are internal or external to the individual.

FIGURE 4.1. THE MOTIVATION PROCESS.

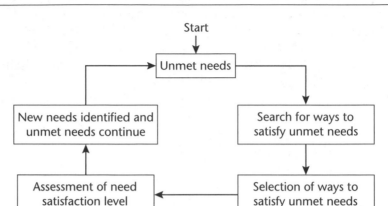

This model also suggests a definition of motivation; motivation is an internal drive that stimulates behavior intended to satisfy an unmet need. In the words of D'Aunno, Fottler, and O'Connor, motivation is "a state of feeling or thinking in which one is energized or aroused to perform a task or engage in a particular behavior" (2000, p. 66). It is important to note that the direction, intensity, and duration of this state can be influenced by outside factors, including the ability of managers to contribute to or impede the satisfaction of the individual's needs.

Motivation is a key determinant of individual performance in work situations and is of obvious importance in accomplishing the desired results established for health programs and projects. However, motivation alone does not fully explain individuals' performance. It is only one of many variables affecting performance. Intelligence, physical and mental abilities, previous experiences, and the nature of the work environment also affect performance. Good equipment and pleasant surroundings facilitate performance. The variables affecting performance can be conceptualized as follows:

$$\text{Performance} = \text{Ability/Talent/Experience} \times \text{Environment} \times \text{Motivation}$$

This equation shows that performance is a function of an interaction of several variables (O'Connor 1998). Without motivation, no amount of ability or talent and no environmental conditions can produce acceptable performance. Although motivation alone will not result in a satisfactory level of performance, it is so central to performance that managers must understand this process if they are to effectively influence the contributions of other participants to achieving a program or project's desired results.

How Motivation Occurs

Because understanding motivation and applying knowledge of how it occurs is so critical to effectively leading others, a great deal of attention has been given to determining the mechanisms of human motivation. To motivate participants, managers need to know the answers to such questions as: What energizes or arouses participants to behave in contributory ways? What variables help direct their energies into particular behaviors? Can the state of arousal be intensified or made to last longer?

It is important to note at the outset that, in seeking answers to questions about motivation, researchers have not established an undisputed and comprehensive theory about motivation or about how managers affect motivation in the workplace. Instead, many competing theories have been posited to explain motivation. These varied approaches to motivation can be divided into two broad categories, *content* perspectives and *process* perspectives (see Figure 4.2). Each of the perspectives contributes something to an understanding of motivation and has implications for the core management activity of leading.

The content perspective on motivation focuses on the internal needs and desires that initiate, sustain, and eventually terminate behavior. The focus is on *what* motivates. In contrast, the process perspective seeks to explain *how* behavior is initiated, sustained, and terminated. Combined, these perspectives on motivation define variables that explain motivated behavior and show how they interact and influence each other to produce certain behavior patterns. Key theories that underpin contemporary thought about human motivation in the workplace are noted in Figure 4.2 and are briefly described in the following sections, beginning with four theories that fall within the content perspective.

Maslow's Hierarchy of Needs. Perhaps the most widely recognized theory about what motivates human behavior—certainly the one with the most enduring impact—was advanced by Abraham Maslow in the 1940s. A psychologist, Maslow formulated a theory of motivation that stressed two fundamental premises (Maslow 1943; 1970). First, he argued that human beings have a variety of needs and that *unmet* needs influence behavior; an adequately fulfilled need is not a motivator. His second premise was that people's needs are arranged in a hierarchy. Maslow stresses the idea of needs existing in a hierarchy, with "higher" needs becoming dominant only after "lower" needs are satisfied. Figure 4.3 illustrates Maslow's needs hierarchy, with examples of each category of need that can be fulfilled in a health program or project.

FIGURE 4.2. COMPARISON OF CONTENT AND PROCESS PERSPECTIVES ON MOTIVATION.

Content Perspective

Focus:

Identifying factors within individuals that initiate, sustain, and terminate behaviors

Key studies:

Maslow's five levels of human needs in hierarchy

Alderfer's three levels of human needs in hierarchy

Herzberg's two sets of factors

McClelland's three learned needs

Implication for managers in leading:

Managers must pay attention to the unique and varied needs, desires, and goals of participants

Process Perspective

Focus:

Explaining how behaviors are initiated, sustained, and terminated

Key studies:

Vroom's expectancy theory of choices

Adams' equity theory

Locke's goal-setting theory

Implication for managers in leading:

Managers must understand how the unique and varied needs, desires, and goals of participants interact with their preferences and with rewards and accomplishments to affect their behavioral choices

FIGURE 4.3. MASLOW'S NEEDS HIERARCHY.

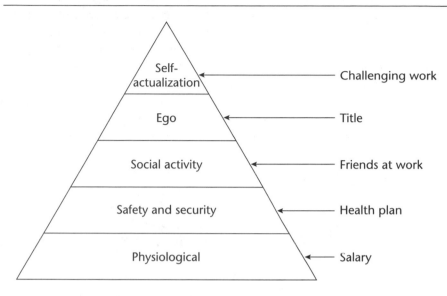

From lowest to highest order, the five categories of needs in Maslow's hierarchy begin with basic physiological needs, such as air, water, food, shelter, and sex, which are necessary for survival. Participants can satisfy many of these needs through the resources that their paychecks provide. After basic physiological needs come safety and security needs. Once survival needs are met, attention can be turned to ensuring continued survival by protecting oneself against physical harm and deprivation. Participants seek to meet their safety and security needs through assuring job security, having adequate life and health insurance, and other benefits. The third level of needs is for social activity, which relates to people's social and gregarious nature, and includes their needs for belonging, friendship, affection, and love. The ability to have friendships with other participants and to engage in social activity within the workplace helps satisfy these needs.

It is important to note that the third-level needs are something of a breaking point in the hierarchy because these needs move away from the physical or quasi-physical needs of the first two levels. This level reflects people's needs for association or companionship, belonging to groups, and for giving and receiving friendship and affection.

The fourth level, ego needs, includes two different types of needs, the need for a positive self-image and for self-respect and the need for recognition and respect from others. Examples of ego needs are the need for independence, achievement, recognition from others, self-esteem, and status. Opportunities for advancement within programs or projects, or within the larger organizations within which they may be embedded, can help participants fulfill these needs.

The top level of the Maslow hierarchy includes self-actualization needs. These fifth-level needs have to do with realizing one's potential for continued growth and development. In effect, these needs represent the need to become everything a person is capable of being. Self-actualization needs are evidenced in people by their need to be creative and to have opportunities for self-expression and self-fulfillment. A challenging and satisfying job is a primary pathway to satisfying such needs in contemporary society.

In part because of its great intuitive appeal, Maslow's concept of what motivates human behavior has been widely adopted. However, in a remarkable bit of candor, he once wrote of his concern that the theory was "being swallowed whole by all sorts of enthusiastic people, who really should be a little more tentative" (Maslow 1965, p. 56). Although this view of what motivates human behavior has limitations, it makes a crucial and valid point that people have numerous needs, which they seek to fulfill. In this way, Maslow contributes important insight into the nature of motivation; his theories account for how unmet needs influence behaviors to fulfill them. Maslow's views on motivation provided a conceptual framework that was used to build and test more sophisticated theories about needs and how they affect human behavior. Two of these theories are described next.

Alderfer's ERG Theory. In another theory of what motivates human behavior, Clayton Alderfer (1969; 1972) advanced the idea that the hierarchy of needs is more accurately conceptualized as having only three distinct categories, not five as in Maslow's formulation. This theory is known as the ERG theory for the three categories of needs, **e**xistence, **r**elatedness, and **g**rowth. Existence needs include material and physical needs that can be satisfied by such things as air, water, money, and working conditions. Relatedness needs include all needs that involve other people. Relatedness needs are satisfied by meaningful social and interpersonal relationships. Growth needs, in Alderfer's scheme, include all needs involving creative efforts. Individuals satisfy these needs through creative or productive contributions.

Alderfer's ERG theory is obviously similar to Maslow's. His existence needs are similar to Maslow's physiological and safety needs; his relatedness needs are similar to Maslow's affection and social activity category; and his growth needs are similar to the self-esteem and self-realization needs that were identified by Maslow. The theories differ, however, in regards to how needs predominate in influencing behavior.

Maslow theorized that unfulfilled lower-level needs are predominant and that the next higher level of needs is not activated until the predominant (unmet lower-level) need is satisfied. He called this the *satisfaction-progression process.* In contrast, Alderfer argued that three categories of needs form a hierarchy only in the sense of increasing abstractness or decreasing concreteness: as an individual moves from existence to relatedness to growth needs, the means to satisfy the needs become less and less concrete.

In Alderfer's theory, people focus first on needs that are satisfied in relatively concrete ways; then they focus on needs that are satisfied more abstractly. This is similar to Maslow's idea of satisfaction-progression. However, Alderfer proposed that a *frustration-regression process* is also present in determining which category of needs predominates at any time. By this he means that someone frustrated in efforts to satisfy growth needs may regress and focus on satisfying more concrete relatedness or even more concrete existence needs. In Alderfer's view, the coexistence of the satisfaction-progression and the frustration-regression processes leads to a *cycling* between categories of needs. A case example from a health program will help to clarify Alderfer's concept of cycling.

Consider the case of Jennifer Smith, a thirty-two-year-old registered nurse who is a participant in a women's health program sponsored by a major hospital. Ms. Smith, a single parent of two children, is appropriately concerned about the security of her position and her pay and benefits, although she finds the social interactions with co-workers rewarding. Clinically, she is an excellent nurse who enjoys her work.

When a vacancy occurs in a nurse manager position in the program, Ms. Smith considers the opportunities this presents for professional growth and development, as well as for a higher salary. She applies for the position and looks forward to the challenges she will face if selected.

However, a more experienced and equally qualified nurse is promoted. Ms. Smith's disappointment shows, and she also becomes quite concerned about her future in the program. Several other participants in the program notice her reaction and make special efforts to ease her disappointment. They tell her that other opportunities will arise, and with more experience she will be promoted.

The newly promoted nurse manager is sensitive to this situation and makes a point of telling Ms. Smith what a valuable contribution she is making to the success of the program. After a few weeks, Ms. Smith returns to the same level of work enjoyment she felt before this episode. In terms of needs, she has *cycled* from having existence and relatedness needs predominate, to focusing on growth needs represented by the promotion, and then returned to relatedness needs, all in a few weeks. In other words, Ms. Smith has experienced a *satisfaction-progression process* and a *frustration-regression process*.

Another important part of Alderfer's ERG theory, and another way in which it differs from Maslow's formulation is Alderfer's view that when individuals satisfy their existence and relatedness needs these needs become less important. The opposite is true for growth needs, however. In Alderfer's view, as growth needs are satisfied they become increasingly important. People who become more creative and productive raise their growth goals and are dissatisfied until the new goals are reached. In the case of Jennifer Smith described previously, this means that when she becomes a nurse manager she will likely raise her goals, anticipating further growth and development in her career.

Herzberg's Two-Factor Theory.   Frederich Herzberg took a different approach to the study of what motivates human behavior in the workplace. He began with questions about what satisfies or dissatisfies people at work, assuming that the answers would contribute to an understanding of what motivates people (Herzberg 1987; Herzberg, Mausner, and Snyderman 1959).

Herzberg and his associates found that one set of factors was associated with satisfaction and high levels of motivation, and another, different set of factors was associated with dissatisfaction and low motivation. Their *two-factor theory* of motivation argues that one set of factors, called *satisfiers* or *motivators,* results in satisfaction and high motivation when present in adequate levels or form. These factors are achievement, recognition, advancement, the work itself, the possibility of growth, and responsibility. The other set of factors, which is labeled *dissatisfiers* or *hygiene factors,* causes dissatisfaction and low motivation when not present in adequate levels or form. These factors include organizational policy and administration, supervision, interpersonal relations, and working conditions.

The most important contribution of Hertzberg's formulation lies in the fact that it has caused managers to think more carefully about the factors that contribute to motivation and about what they can do to enhance opportunities for people to achieve intrinsic satisfaction from their work. If managers are to help participants be motivated, they must be concerned with one set of factors to minimize dissatisfaction and another set of factors to help participants achieve satisfaction and be motivated in their work.

McClelland's Learned Needs Theory.   Another important contributor to the content perspective of motivation was David McClelland (1961; 1975; 1985), who developed the *learned needs theory.* McClelland posits that people learn some of their needs through life experiences; they are not born with the needs. This theory builds on the much earlier work of Murray (1938) who theorized that people acquire an individual profile of needs by interacting with their environment. McClelland was also influenced by the work of Atkinson (1961) and Atkinson and Raynor (1974).

Both McClelland and Atkinson argue that people have three distinct sets of needs: (1) the need for achievement, including the need to excel, achieve in relation to standards, accomplish complex tasks, and resolve problems; (2) the need for power, including the need to control or influence how others behave and to exercise authority over others; and (3) the need for affiliation, including the need to associate with others, to form and sustain friendly and close interpersonal relationships, and to avoid conflict.

McClelland hypothesized that people are not born with these needs. Instead, these needs are *learned* or acquired as people grow and develop. For example, children learn the need to achieve in part through encouragement and rewards for performance in academic and sports activities by adults who influence their early years.

McClelland also posits that everyone has these three sets of needs, although one predominates and most strongly affects each individual's behavior. This point is important because it relates to how well people fit into particular work situations. In fact, the most useful aspect of McClelland's formulation is the importance of matching a person's particular dominant needs with the work situation. If this is done carefully, participants will be more motivated and their performance will reflect this.

The content perspective on motivation, as reflected in the four theories or models discussed previously, emphasizes that human motivation originates from the needs of people and their search to satisfy these needs. The common thread running through the content models is their focus on needs that motivate human behavior. Each theory defines human needs differently, but all support the concept that managers can help motivate participants in their programs and projects by helping them identify their specific needs and at least, in part, meet the needs in the workplace.

These models emphasize the importance of managers helping participants understand their needs and helping them find ways to satisfy the needs within the workplace. These are extraordinarily complex tasks in view of the fact that each person has a unique and constantly changing set of needs. Managers can help participants identify and meet their needs by empathizing with them. Combining empathy with effective two-way communication, as discussed in Chapter Six, usually results in progress toward identifying and fulfilling needs.

The content theories of motivation with their singular focus on what motivates behavior provide many useful insights for managers. However, other models are needed to provide insight into the process of motivation, to explain the mechanisms through which motivation occurs. The process perspective focuses on how individuals' expectations and preferences for outcomes that are associated with or that result from their performance actually influence performance. A central element in the process perspective on motivation is that people are decision makers who weigh the personal advantages and disadvantages of their behaviors.

Continuing to follow the outline presented in Figure 4.2, three theories that fall within the process perspective on motivation are briefly presented next: *Vroom's expectancy theory, Adams's equity theory,* and *Locke's goal-setting theory.* These are the major models of the processes by which motivation occurs; each model seeks to explain how motivation occurs in human beings.

Vroom's Expectancy Theory. Victor Vroom's formulation of how motivation occurs is based on the idea that, although people are driven by their unmet needs, they make decisions about how they will and will not behave in attempting to fulfill their needs. Their decisions are affected by three conditions: (1) people must believe that through their own efforts they are more likely to achieve desired levels of performance, (2) people must believe that achieving the desired level of performance will lead to some concrete outcome or reward, and (3) people must value the outcome (Vroom 1964). Figure 4.4 shows the three central components and the relationships in the expectancy theory model.

In this model, *expectancy* is what individuals perceive to be the probability that their efforts will lead to desired levels of performance. If a person believes that more effort will lead to improved performance, expectancy will be high. If, in a different situation, the same person believes that trying harder will not improve performance, the expectancy will be low.

FIGURE 4.4. BASIC MODEL OF EXPECTANCY THEORY.

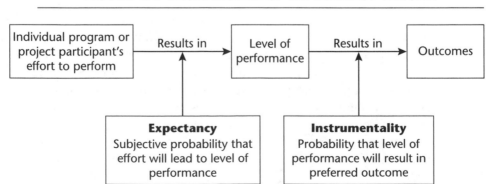

Instrumentality is the probability perceived by individuals that their performance will lead to desired outcomes or rewards. If a person believes that better performance will be rewarded, the instrumentality of performance to reward will be high. Conversely, if the person believes that improved performance will not be rewarded, the instrumentality of improved performance will be low.

Outcomes are listed only once in Figure 4.4, but they play two important roles in the expectancy theory. *Level of performance* (in the center of Figure 4.4) actually represents an *outcome* of the *individual effort to perform* component of the figure. Vroom calls this a first-order outcome. Examples of first-order outcomes include productivity, creativity, absenteeism, quality of work, or other behaviors that result from an individual's effort to perform. The outcomes component shown on the right side of Figure 4.4 is a second-order outcome that results from attainment of first-order outcomes. That is, these outcomes are the rewards (or punishments) associated with performance. Examples include merit pay increases, esteem of co-workers, approval of the program or project's manager, promotion, and flexible work schedules.

Crucial to Vroom's expectancy theory is the concept that people have preferences for outcomes. Vroom termed the value an individual attaches to a particular outcome its *valence*. When an individual has a strong preference for a particular outcome it receives a high valence; similarly, a lower preference for an outcome yields a lower valence. People have valences for both first- and second-order outcomes. For example, a participant in a program or project might prefer a merit pay increase to a flexible work schedule, while another participant prefers the flexibility (second-order outcomes). A participant might prefer to produce quality work (a first-order outcome) because this person believes quality work will lead to a merit pay increase (a second-order outcome).

The three components of the expectancy theory (expectancy, instrumentality, and valence for outcomes) can be combined into an equation to express the motivation to work:

$$\text{Motivation} = \text{Expectancy} \times \text{Instrumentality} \times \text{Valence}$$

$$\text{or}$$

$$M = E \times I \times V$$

It is important to note that because the equation is multiplicative, a low value assigned to any variable will yield a low result. For example, if a person is certain that effort will lead to performance, an Expectancy value of 1.0 is assigned. If a person is certain that performance will lead to reward, an Instrumentality value of 1.0 is assigned. And if a person does not have a very high valence or preference for the reward involved, a Valence value of 0.5 is assigned. When multiplied $(1.0 \times 1.0 \times 0.5 = 0.5)$, the result is low, indicating that motivation is low. For motivation to be high, expectancy, instrumentality, and valence values all must be high.

For managers of programs and projects, expectancy theory explains a great deal about motivated behavior. By applying expectancy theory, managers focus on leverage points that help them influence the motivation of other participants. For motivated behavior to occur, three conditions must be met: (1) the participant must have a high expectancy that effort and performance are actually linked, (2) the participant must have a high expectancy that performance will lead to outcomes or rewards, and (3) the participant must assign a high valence value (have a preference) to the outcomes that result from effort, including both first- and second-order outcomes.

Managers who know what participants prefer in terms of second-order outcomes for their efforts and performance have an advantage in developing effective approaches to their motivation. It is important to remember that implicit in Vroom's model is the fact that individuals have different preferences about outcomes. The design of approaches to motivation must reflect this fact; the approaches must be flexible enough to address differences in individual preferences regarding the rewards of work.

Bateman and Zeithaml (1993) identify three crucial implications for management work inherent in expectancy theory. First, they argue that managers should take steps to increase expectancies. This means providing a work environment that facilitates work performance and establishing realistic performance objectives. It also means providing training, support, and encouragement at levels that permit participants to be confident they can perform their work at the levels expected of them.

Second, Bateman and Zeithaml urge managers to identify positively valent outcomes for participants they seek to motivate. This means thinking about what jobs provide to those who occupy them, as well as what is not provided by these jobs, but could be. Managers must think about how and why different participants assign different valences to outcomes and what this means for motivating behavior. In considering outcomes with positive valences for participants, managers must think about the needs participants seek to fulfill through work.

Third, Bateman and Zeithaml stress that managers make performance instrumental to positive outcomes. Managers can do this, for example, by making certain that good performance is followed by such positive results as praise and recognition, by favorable performance reviews, pay increases, or other positive results. Conversely, managers should make certain that poor performance has fewer positive outcomes and more negative ones than does good performance. Instrumentality, in the context of expectancy theory, means that there is a perceived relationship between performance and outcome, positive or negative.

Adams's Equity Theory. An important extension of expectancy theory arose from the realization that, in addition to preferences as to the outcomes or rewards associated with performance, individuals also assess the degree to which potential rewards will be equitably distributed. Equity theory posits that people calculate the ratios of their efforts to the rewards they receive and compare them to the ratios they believe exist for others in similar situations. They do this because they have a strong desire to be treated fairly. J. Stacy Adams (1963; 1965) argues that people judge equity with the following equation:

$$\frac{O_p}{I_p} = \frac{O_o}{I_o}$$

Where

O_p is the person's perception of the outcomes received

I_p is the person's perception of personal inputs

O_o is the person's perception of the outcomes that a comparison person (or comparison other) is receiving

I_o is the person's perception of the inputs of the comparison person (or comparison other

This formula suggests participants believe equity exists when the perception of the ratio of inputs (efforts) to outcomes (rewards) received is equivalent to that of some *comparison other* or *referent*. Conversely, inequity exists when the ratios are not equivalent.

It is noteworthy that perception, not reality, is considered in this equation. Furthermore, there are options as to the comparison others or referents in the equation, including the following:

- People in similar circumstances (co-workers or someone whose circumstances are thought to be similar)
- A group of people in similar circumstances (for example, all registered nurses working in a particular health program or project)
- The perceiving person under different circumstances (for example, earlier in the person's present position or when they previously occupied another position)

Choice of referent is a function of available information about the options as well as perceived relevance of the options to a particular situation. Finally, it is important to note that in the equation there may be many different inputs and outcomes. Inputs are what people believe they contribute to their jobs and include experience, time, effort, dedication, intelligence, and the like. Outcomes are what people believe they get from their jobs and include pay, promotion, status, esteem, monotony, fatigue, danger, and the like.

Equity theory recognizes that people are concerned both with the absolute rewards they receive for their efforts and with the relationship of these rewards to what others receive. Participants in programs and projects routinely make judgments about the relationship between their inputs and outcomes and the inputs and outcomes of others. In effect, equity theory recognizes that people are interested in distributive fairness—that is, in getting what they believe they deserve for their work. Extensive research reveals that, even with all the variables involved in making comparisons, people regularly consider equity (Walster, Walster, and Berscheid 1978; Mowday 1987); that is, they consistently compare how fairly they are being treated with how fairly they believe others are being treated.

When faced with situations they perceive to be inequitable, people seek to restore equity in a number of different ways. Their alternatives are contained in the equity equation shown previously. They might use some or all of these alternatives simultaneously or in sequence before a feeling of equity is restored or attained. Using pay as an example of something about which equity is important, people who feel an inequity (such as that their pay is too low or that they work harder than others with the same pay) can decrease their input by reducing effort to compensate for this perceived inequity. Alternatively, they could seek to change their total compensation package as a means to reduce the perceived pay inequity. They could seek to modify their comparisons or referents. For example, they might try to persuade low performers who are receiving equal pay to increase their efforts, or they might try to discourage high performers from exerting so much effort.

Others, feeling an inequity in their pay, perhaps in desperation, might distort reality and rationalize that the perceived inequities are somehow justified. As a last resort, people might even choose to leave an inequitable situation. This action usually occurs only when people conclude that the inequities will not be resolved. Thus, participants in a program or project can attempt to restore equity by changing the reality or the perception of the inputs and outcomes in the equity equation. However, each mechanism they use for this purpose can create serious problems for managers.

Equity theory makes an important contribution to understanding human motivation because it shows that motivation is significantly influenced by both absolute and relative rewards. It also shows that if people perceive inequity they act to reduce it. Thus, it is important that managers minimize inequities—real and perceived—in their programs and projects. This means helping participants understand the differences among jobs and the associated rewards, and making

certain that reward differences actually reflect different performance requirements among jobs.

The bottom-line implication of equity theory for managers is that people
who feel equitably treated in their workplaces are more satisfied than those who
feel inequitably treated. Although satisfaction alone does not ensure high levels
of work performance, dissatisfaction, especially when many participants feel it
in a work situation, has very negative consequences, including the following:

- Higher absenteeism and turnover rates
- Lower citizenship behaviors
- More grievances and lawsuits related to the work situation
- Stealing
- Sabotage
- Vandalism
- More job stress
- Other costly negative consequences for health programs and projects and the
  participants in them

The equity theory emphasizes the importance of managers treating the other
participants in their programs and projects fairly.

Locke's Goal-Setting Theory. A third and increasingly popular model within the
process perspective on motivation derives from the work of Edwin Locke (1968;
1969; 1987). Building on the pervasiveness of the goal-directedness of human behavior, Locke viewed goal setting as a cognitive process through which conscious
goals, as well as intentions about pursuing goals, are developed and become
primary determinants of behavior (Wood and Locke 1990).

In Locke's view an important part of motivation in individuals is the intent
to work toward their goals. The central premise in this perspective on the process
of motivation is that people focus their attention on the concrete tasks related
to attaining their goals and persist in the tasks until the goals are achieved
(Latham and Locke 1987; Locke and Latham 1990; Muchinsky 2000).

In general, studies affirm the importance of goals in motivation (Mento, Steel,
and Karren 1987). Locke's original theory that *goal specificity* (the degree of quantitative precision of the goal) and *goal difficulty* (the level of performance required
to reach the goal) are important to motivation has been affirmed by other studies (Naylor and Ilgen 1984). It is also well established that highly specific goals
lead to improvement in individuals' performances because such goals help people to understand what is to be done (Latham and Baldes 1975). Finally, understanding the role of goals in motivation has been enhanced by research that

shows the positive relationship of goal acceptance by a person to that person's performance (Erez and Kanfer 1983). Other studies show that people are more likely to accept goals (other than those they set for themselves), especially difficult goals, when they participate in establishing them (Erez, Earley, and Hulin 1985; Schwartz 1990).

Goals that can effectively motivate desirable behaviors in the workplace have certain characteristics that should be kept in mind as managers set goals for participants in their programs or projects, or as managers encourage participants to set goals for themselves. The most important characteristic of goals, in terms of their ability to motivate, is that goals be acceptable to the people managers wish to help motivate. Acceptability is increased when work-related goals do not conflict with personal values and when people have clear reasons to pursue the goals. It is also important that goals be challenging but attainable, and that they be specific, quantifiable, and measurable (Bateman and Zeithaml 1993). It is also important for managers to provide participants with timely and specific feedback on their progress toward achieving established goals.

Locke's original work and other studies that it stimulated have important implications for managers in health programs and projects. Many of the most significant challenges of leading and of helping participants be motivated in the workplace arise because managers do not clearly define and specify the desired results (outputs, outcomes, and impact) toward which they want participants to contribute. Leading effectively, and using motivation to support this, depends upon clear statements of desired results, to which all participants can link their work-related goals. This is true whether participants establish the goals for themselves or managers either establish the goals for them or establish them in consultation with participants. Statements of desired results are especially useful in motivating behaviors and in leading in general when those who will be influenced by the statements participate in and agree with their formulation.

Conclusion about the Role of Motivation in Leading

The *content* and *process* perspectives on motivation as expressed in the theories and models of motivation discussed previously have guided researchers in their search for answers to the questions of *what* motivates human behaviors and of *how* motivation occurs. Understanding of motivation supports a manager's core activity of leading because leading effectively means *influencing* participants to contribute to achieving a program or project's desired results. Motivation is a means to the end of leading (influencing) participants to make contributions that help accomplish the desired results established for a program or project. Helping motivate participants is not, however, the only means available to managers for use in influencing participants.

Influence and Leading, Interpersonal Power and Influence

We have defined leading by managers as influencing others to understand and agree about what needs to be done in order to achieve the desired results established for a program or project, *and* facilitating the individual and collective contributions of others to achieving the desired results. Because the essence of leading is the ability to influence others, one must fully understand influencing in order to fully understand leading. As discussed in the previous section, motivation is important to the exertion of such influence. However, there is more to influencing than motivation.

In order to fully understand the influence a manager can have over other participants in a program or project, one must first understand *interpersonal power* because interpersonal power is defined as the potential to exert influence over others. Having more interpersonal power translates into having more potential to influence others.

Managers are able to exert influence in the workplace because they have interpersonal power. To a great extent, managers have interpersonal power in work settings because they are managers. It may be useful to review the discussion of authority in Chapter Three, where it is noted that the most important source of a manager's interpersonal power is the formal position the manager holds in a program or project's organization design. This is the formal power or authority assigned to managers in organization designs to support their ability to manage effectively.

All program and project managers have some degree of interpersonal power or authority based on their position. Of course, managers at different hierarchical levels within organization designs have different amounts of positional interpersonal power. Positional power permits managers to exert influence by control over rewards that can be used to support motivation, or to coerce participants.

Managers have significant interpersonal power that derives from the following:

- Their control over certain aspects of the physical environment in which work occurs.
- Their ability to shape elements of a program or project's logic model, including determination of desired results, processes used, and inputs/resources available (see Figure 1.1).
- Their role in establishing the organization design for a program or project. When managers design work flow arrangements, for example, they can determine which participants interact with others, or who initiates a linked series of actions. Similarly, their ability to cluster certain individual positions into units, to assign reporting relationships, or to design information systems are position-based sources of managers' interpersonal power.

Control over information is a source of interpersonal power in any organizational setting. To a great extent, this source of interpersonal power is positional. Managers have access to certain information because of their positions in organizational designs. To have interpersonal power derived from control over information, a person must actively cultivate a network of information sources. Cultivation of this network is influenced by a manager's position in an organization design.

Another aspect of a manager's interpersonal power is that such power can be acquired by a manager's possession and use of political skills. Interpersonal power can derive from control over key decisions, ability to form coalitions, ability to co-opt or diffuse and weaken the influence of rivals, and ability to institutionalize the manager's power by exploiting ambiguity to interpret events in a manner favorable to the manager (Yukl 2002). Position can help a manager use political skill, but the skill is inherent in the manager. This illustrates a second important source of interpersonal power, the characteristics and attributes of the person with the interpersonal power.

The existence of interpersonal power in work settings that is based upon what an individual knows or is able to do has been recognized for many years. It has been called *expert power* (French and Raven 1959). This is power determined by a person possessing knowledge that is valued by the program or project or by the larger organization in which it is embedded. Thus, expert power is different from *positional interpersonal power,* which is primarily determined by a manager's position in the organization design. Any participant in a program or project can possess expert power. For example, physicians or nurses whose expertise is vital to the success of a program or project possess interpersonal power. Power based on expertise is not limited to those in particular positions in organization designs.

Another source of interpersonal power, sometimes called charismatic power, or referent power (French and Raven 1959), results when one individual engenders admiration, loyalty, and emulation to the extent that it permits the person to influence others. As with power based on expertise, referent power cannot be assigned to a person based on position in an organization design. Referent power is typically developed only over a long period of close interaction in which a person, who may or may not be a manager, demonstrates friendliness, concern for the needs and feelings of others, and fairness toward them. It is rare for a leader to gain sufficient power to heavily influence followers simply from referent or charismatic power.

Managers in all programs and projects have multiple sources or bases of interpersonal power, although managers' have different levels of power based on the sources available to them. For example, one manager may have interpersonal power because of formal positional authority over the program or project and its participants. This manager may have some degree of control over inputs/resources, rewards, punishments, and information and may have more relevant expertise in the work of the program or project than others. Yet he may possess little power based on political skill.

Another manager may derive interpersonal power from the same menu of sources, but in a different mix. For example, this manager may possess an exceptional level of political power by virtue of authority to control decision processes, the ability to form coalitions of key internal and external stakeholders, or the ability to co-opt opponents. Still another manager may have considerable charisma, extremely loyal participants in the program or project, and personal friendships with key leaders of the organization in which it is embedded, all of which provide this manager with considerable interpersonal power.

Certainly, the possession of interpersonal power derived from some mix of the sources noted previously is an important precursor to exerting influence over others or to leading them effectively. But alone, interpersonal power does not explain influence or leading. Interpersonal power, as noted previously, is the *potential* to exert influence. How does one manager convert interpersonal power, from whatever sources, into influence, while another manager with equal power is unable to convert interpersonal power to influence? The search for answers to this question has been an evolutionary process, resulting in a better understanding of leading.

The Ongoing Search to Understand Effective Leading

During the last century, researchers have used three general approaches to understand how effective leading is accomplished in work settings. The *traits approach* is based on the proposition that traits, skills, abilities, or characteristics inherent in some people explain why they are more effective at leading than others. The *behaviors approach,* which grew directly out of the inability of traits to fully explain effective leading, is based on the assumption that particular behaviors or sets of behaviors that make up a style of leading might be associated with success in leading. A third approach, called the *situational approach,* integrates the traits and behaviors approaches by arguing that traits and behaviors must be combined with particular situations to explain effective leading. Figure 4.5 summarizes the evolutionary relationships these three approaches bear to one another. Key insights drawn from studies conducted within each approach are described in the following sections.

FIGURE 4.5. COMPARING THREE APPROACHES TO UNDERSTANDING EFFECTIVE LEADING.

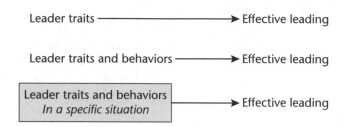

Leader Traits

The earliest studies of leading were based on the idea that particular physical or personality traits distinguish effective leaders. In attempting to prove the so-called trait theory of leadership, researchers sought to find traits that all effective leaders possessed. Many different traits were studied, including physical characteristics such as height, weight, and appearance, and personality traits such as alertness, originality, integrity, and self-confidence, as well as intelligence or cleverness. Although the search for universal leader traits was not fruitful (Stogdill 1948; 1974), researchers have identified traits and patterns of traits that tend to be associated with effective leaders.

Although research shows that possession of certain traits alone does not guarantee leadership success, there is evidence that effective leaders are different from other people in certain key respects. Key leader traits include

- Drive (a broad term which includes achievement, motivation, ambition, energy, tenacity, and initiative)
- Leadership motivation (the desire to lead but not to seek power as an end in itself)
- Honesty and integrity
- Self-confidence (which is associated with emotional stability)
- Cognitive ability
- Knowledge

There is less clear evidence for traits such as charisma, creativity, and flexibility (Kirkpatrick and Locke 1991, p. 48).

Goleman (1995; 1998) finds an association between what he terms a leader's *emotional intelligence* and effectiveness at leading. He identifies five components of emotional intelligence: self-awareness, self-regulation, motivation, empathy, and social skill. Self-awareness is the ability to recognize one's own moods, emotions, and drives as well as to determine their effect on others. Self-regulation refers to the ability to control or redirect negative or disruptive moods or emotions. Motivation, in Goleman's view, reflects a strong drive to achieve and to pursue desired results with energy and persistence. Empathy means the ability to understand other people. Social skill refers to being proficient in building relationships and to being persuasive. Goleman argues that without emotional intelligence, "a person can have the best training in the world, an incisive, analytical mind, and an endless supply of smart ideas, but still won't make a great leader" (1998, p. 94).

As researchers expanded their perspectives on the role of leader traits in effectiveness at leading, some of them came to view traits as predispositions to *behaviors*. They adopted the view that "A particular trait, or set of them, tends to predispose (although does not cause) an individual to engage in certain behaviors that may or may not result in leadership effectiveness" (Pointer and Sanchez 2000, p. 111). These researchers began to appreciate that traits had an impact on effectiveness at leading, but not in the way imagined in the earlier search for universal traits of leaders. They came to understand that "What seems to be most important is not traits but rather how they are expressed in the behavior of the leader" (Van Fleet and Yukl 1989, p. 67), or in the broader concept of *leadership style*.

Leader Behaviors and Styles of Leading

Studies of the relationships between behaviors and styles of leading exhibited by leaders and their effectiveness was premised on the exciting possibility that, if especially successful behaviors or styles could be identified, then people could be taught how to be leaders. Leaders would not have to be born with certain traits or attributes. The ensuing studies in leader behavior focused on describing leader behaviors, on developing concepts and models of styles of leading (styles being thought of as combinations of behaviors), and on examining the relationships between styles and effectiveness in leading. These studies added an important dimension to the understanding of leading and new insights into effectiveness in leading.

The most important early studies of leader behaviors were conducted in the late 1940s at Ohio State University and at the University of Michigan. In fact, most studies of leader behavior are based, at least in part, on this pioneering work. The Ohio State University studies identified two dimensions of leader behavior, *consideration* and *initiating structure* (Stogdill and Coons 1957).

Consideration was defined as the degree to which a leader acts in a friendly and supportive manner, shows concern for followers, and looks out for their welfare. Initiating structure was defined as the degree to which a leader defines and structures the work to be done by followers and the extent to which attention was focused on achieving desired results established by the leader. These dimensions were not viewed as ends of a spectrum of behavior, but as two distinct and separate dimensions.

Other researchers at the University of Michigan paralleled the studies at Ohio State University. Based on extensive interviews of leaders and followers in a variety of organizations, Likert and his colleagues at Michigan identified two distinct styles of leader behavior, *job-centered* and *employee-centered* (Likert 1961). In these studies, leaders who were employee-centered emphasized interpersonal relations, took a personal interest in the needs of their subordinates, and readily accepted differences among work group members. These leaders were considerate, supportive, and helpful with followers.

In contrast, job-centered leaders emphasized technical or task aspects of the job, were more concerned with participants accomplishing their tasks than anything else, and regarded participants as a means to this end. These leaders spent their time planning, scheduling, coordinating, and closely supervising the work of participants.

Studies conducted in a variety of settings found that effective leaders were employee-centered and focused on the needs of the participants. These studies also demonstrated that, in addition to being employee-centered, effective leaders established high performance objectives for participants but permitted them to participate in establishing the objectives (Katz and Kahn 1952; 1978).

Likert, who was especially influenced by the findings on employee-centered behaviors, came to believe that a key element in effective leadership was the degree to which leaders allow followers to influence the leader's decisions. He believed that participation encourages acceptance of decisions and commitment to them, both of which contribute directly to productivity and to follower satisfaction (Likert 1977). His views on the benefits of participatory leadership stimulated substantial research on its effects. Miller and Monge (1986) provide a good meta-analytic review of studies of the value of participatory leadership. The relevance of these studies to managing health programs and projects can be summarized as follows:

- Participation encourages participants to identify more closely with the program or project. This enhances motivation, especially regarding such contributory behaviors as cooperation, protecting fellow participants and property, avoiding waste, and generally going beyond the call of duty. If people have a voice in their work, they tend to be more enthusiastic in performing the work.

- Participation can be a means to overcome resistance to change. Those who participate in decisions about change will have a better understanding of the need for change and be less likely to resist change.
- Participation enhances the personal growth and development of a program or project's participants. By participating in decisions, participants gain experience and become more proficient in decision making.
- Participation enables a wider range of ideas and experiences to be brought to bear on a problem or opportunity. Often participants who are closer to a situation and more familiar with it can develop ideas as to how to solve problems or take advantage of opportunities more readily than managers.
- Participation increases flexibility within how a program or project's logic model works because participants gain a wider range of experience about how its various components (see Figure 1.1) fit together and work.

The behavioral studies provided the intellectual foundation for subsequent efforts to identify effective styles of leading by identifying the optimal mix of leadership behaviors to achieve effectiveness. (Remember that styles of leading mean particular combinations of behaviors.) One such effort that has been useful for depicting variations in leadership styles was undertaken by Blake and Mouton (1985) and subsequently expanded by Blake and McCanse (1991). Their model of leader styles uses two variables—concern for people and concern for production—as the axes of a diagram on which they plot styles.

The people orientation focuses on enhancing the leader's relationships with followers. The production orientation focuses on tasks and objectives in relation to performing work. The two orientations can be used to create a diagram to help visualize the variation in possible styles of leading. For example, using a scale from 1 (minimum concern) to 10 (maximum concern), a style characterized by minimum concern for both people and production would be located at the bottom left side of the diagram. Similarly, a maximum concern for people and for production would be located at the top right of the diagram. Different levels of concern for these two variables permit plotting of various styles of leading.

Tannenbaum and Schmidt (1973) developed a model in which several possible styles of leading are arrayed as a continuum. This model shows alternative styles based upon how much participation leaders permit other participants in their decision making. The resulting styles of leading, with the labels given them by Tannenbaum and Schmidt, are as follows:

- *Autocratic leaders* make decisions and announce them to other participants. The role of other participants is to carry out orders without an opportunity to materially alter decisions already made by the manager.

- *Consultative leaders* convince other participants of the correctness of the decision by carefully explaining the rationale for the decision and its effect on the other participants and on the program or project. A second consultative style is practiced when managers permit slightly more involvement by other participants. For example, the manager might present decisions to other participants and also invite questions to enhance understanding and acceptance.
- *Participative leaders* present tentative decisions that will be changed if other participants can make a convincing case for a different decision. A second participative style is practiced when a manager presents a problem to participants, seeks their advice and suggestions, but then makes the decision. This style of leading makes greater use of participation and less use of authority than do autocratic and consultative styles.
- *Democratic leaders* define the limits of the situation and problem to be solved and permit other participants to make the decision.
- *Laissez-faire leaders* permit other participants to have great discretion in decision making. The manager participates in decision making with no more influence than other participants. Leaders' and other participants' roles in decision making are indistinguishable in this style.

The importance of the Tannenbaum and Schmidt model to understanding leading lies in their conclusion that the best style of leading depends on the circumstances present in a particular situation. In their view, the choice of a style should be based on the following factors:

- The manager's value system, confidence in other participants, and tolerance for ambiguity and uncertainty
- Factors within the other participants in a situation, such as their expectations, need for independence, ability, knowledge, and experience
- Factors in the particular situation, such as the logic model, organization design, nature of the problem to be solved or the work to be done, and time pressure

Tannenbaum and Schmidt made a significant leap forward in understanding leading by arguing that no single style of leading is correct all of the time or in all situations. Leaders must adapt and change styles to fit different situations. An autocratic style might be appropriate in certain clinical situations in programs and projects where work frequently involves a high degree of urgency. However, this style could be disastrous in other situations. The Tannenbaum and Schmidt model identifies a set of relatively discrete styles of leading but couples these different styles with the concept that certain factors dictate choosing one style over the others. The factors noted previously include some that are internal to the manager, some that are internal to the other participants, and some that relate to the particular situation. In this way, Tannenbaum and Schmidt's model provides a bridge between the early trait and behavioral studies of leading and contemporary—and much more sophisticated—*situational* or *contingency models* of leading that are described in the next section.

Situational or Contingency Models of Leading

When it was found that effectiveness of leading could not be fully explained by traits, behaviors, or styles, and especially when it was found that behaviors and styles appropriate and effective in one situation produced failure in others, researchers turned their attention to incorporating situational influences, or contingencies, into models of leading. From among the many resulting models that seek to explain how situational variables help to determine the relative effectiveness of leading styles, three of the most important are described briefly. The path-goal model developed by IIouse and Mitchell (1974) is given most attention because it is the most useful of the situational models.

Fiedler's Contingency Model. Fred Fiedler (1964; 1967) sought to specify situations in which certain leader traits are especially effective. His hypothesis was that effective leading is contingent upon whether the elements in a particular leading situation fit specific traits of the leader. Complex theories leave ample room for criticism and Fiedler's is no exception. Considerable research, however, supports the model (Peters, Hartke, and Pohlman 1985).

Fiedler's work is important because it represents the first comprehensive attempt to incorporate situational variables directly into a model of leading. This new dimension was refined in many subsequent studies. The contingency model has utility in management practice, especially in suggesting to managers the importance of systematically assessing whether their interpersonal relationships with participants in their programs and projects are supportive of the participants. The contingency model also considers how the organization designs and processes being used fit managers' leading styles.

Hershey and Blanchard's Situational Model. Paul Hershey and Kenneth Blanchard (1996) developed a model of leading that attempts to explain leading effectiveness as interplay among: (1) The manager's relationship behavior, defined as the extent to which managers maintain personal relationships with other participants through open communication and by exhibiting supportive behaviors and actions toward them, (2) The manager's task behavior, which is the extent to which managers organize and define the roles of participants and guide and direct them, and (3) The participants' readiness level, by which Hershey and Blanchard mean their readiness to perform a task or function or to pursue a particular goal.

This model focuses on those participants a manager is attempting to lead as the most important situational variable and specifically focuses on participants' readiness to perform. The central premise is that appropriate leading style depends on the readiness level of the people the manager is seeking to influence. In this model, readiness is assessed by two factors, ability and willingness. Ability refers to the knowledge, experience, and skill that an individual or group possesses. Willingness is the extent to which an individual or group has the commitment and motivation needed to accomplish a specific task.

The Hershey and Blanchard model is widely used by managers and emphasizes several important aspects of leader behavior in determining effectiveness in leading. Managers engaged in leading must be concerned about the readiness of other participants to be led, and they must recognize that managers can affect the level of readiness of other participants. This model also provides a useful reminder to managers that it is important to treat all participants in a program or project as individuals, with real differences among them. Moreover, the model reminds managers to treat the same participant differently over time, as the participant changes in terms of readiness level (Bateman and Zeithaml 1993).

House's Path-Goal Model of Leading. Like the other situational or contingency models of leading described previously, the path-goal model attempts to predict the leader behaviors that will be most effective in particular situations. This model is perhaps the most generally useful situational model of leading effectiveness. Its name is derived from its focus on how leaders influence participants' perceptions of their work goals and the paths they follow toward attaining these goals. Robert House, in the original conception of this model, posited that the leader's functions are to increase the personal payoffs to followers for attaining their work-related goals and to make the path to these payoffs smoother (House 1971). House and Terence Mitchell, who helped develop the theory further, believe that "leaders are effective because of their impact on subordinates' motivation, ability to perform effectively, and satisfaction" (House and Mitchell 1974, p. 81). This theory is called path-goal because it focuses on how leaders influence their subordinates' perceptions of the subordinates' work goals, personal goals, and paths to goal attainment. The path-goal theory incorporates the concept that leader behaviors are motivating or satisfying to the degree that the behaviors increase subordinates' goal attainment and clarifies the paths to attaining these goals (House and Mitchell 1974).

This model of leading relies on the results of the Ohio State University and the University of Michigan leadership studies and on the previously described expectancy theory of motivation. The expectancy model focuses on describing the relationships among expectancy, instrumentality, and valence. Expectancy is the perceived probability that effort will affect performance. (Instrumentality is the perceived probability that performance will lead to outcomes. Valence is the value attached to an outcome by a person.) The path-goal model of leadership focuses on the factors that affect expectancy, instrumentality, and valence. Leaders can increase the valences associated with work-goal attainment, the instrumentalities of work-goal attainment, and the expectancy that effort will result in work-goal attainment.

The path-goal model is situational because its basic premise is that the effect of leader behavior on follower performance and satisfaction depends on the situation, specifically upon follower characteristics and work characteristics. Stated in another way, different leadership behaviors are best for different situations. According to House and Mitchell (1974), there are four categories of leader behavior, each of which is best suited to a particular situation:

1. *Directive leading* describes the behavior of the leader who tells followers what they must do, tells them how to do it, requires they follow rules and procedures, and schedules and coordinates the work.
2. *Supportive leading* describes the behavior of the leader who is friendly and approachable and exhibits consideration for the well-being and needs of followers.
3. *Participative leading* describes the behavior of the leader who consults with followers, asks for opinions and suggestions, and considers them.
4. *Achievement-oriented leading* describes the behavior of the leader who establishes challenging goals for followers, expects excellent performance, and exhibits confidence they will meet expectations.

House believes all four styles of leader behavior can and should be used by leaders as the situation dictates and that effective leaders match styles to situations. Situations can vary along two dimensions. One dimension is the nature of the people being led. Followers may or may not have the ability to do the job. They differ, too, as to the perceived degree of control they have over their work. The second dimension is the nature of the task, which may be routine and one with which followers have prior experience—or it may be new and ambiguous and one that requires help.

The path-goal model shows that effective leaders diagnose the situation and match behavior to it. For example, directive leading could be used when followers are not well trained for their work and the work they are doing is partly routine and partly ambiguous. Supportive or participative leading might be most appropriate if followers are doing highly routine work and have experience with this work. Achievement-oriented leading would be effective if followers are doing highly innovative and ambiguous work and if they have high levels of work-related knowledge and skill, conditions often found in health programs and projects.

The path-goal model of leading, in its essence, suggests that managers in programs and projects improve leading effectiveness by: (1) Making the path to achieving work goals easier by providing coaching and direction for participants when needed, (2) removing or minimizing frustrating barriers that interfere with participants' abilities to achieve work goals, and (3) increasing the payoffs for participants when they achieve work-related goals.

House and Mitchell's path-goal model is a useful construct because it merges concepts and knowledge of motivating and leading. The model also provides a pragmatic framework that is valuable to managers as they seek to match their leader behaviors to characteristics of the participants they seek to lead, as well as to characteristics of the logic models and organization designs of their programs and projects.

Toward an Integrative Approach to Effective Leading

Clearly, managers' effectiveness at leading contributes to the performance of individual participants, teams, and work groups, as well as to entire programs and projects. Among the core activities of managers, effective leading is as important as effective strategizing and designing.

Three approaches to understanding leading–traits, behaviors, and situational or contingency approaches (see Figure 4.5)–have been presented. These different approaches have resulted in numerous models, each seeking to explain the phenomenon of effective leading. Individually, however, none of the models fully explains how a leader is effective. Levey suggests, "We will probably never be able to achieve a truly elegant and rigorous general theory of leadership" (1990, p. 479). This view reflects the complexity and variety of variables involved in leading. Leading is a dynamic process "that does not reside solely within a given person or a given situation; rather, situations create an interplay of needs, and effective leaders work to continually identify and meet them" (Druskat and Wheeler 2003, p. 438).

It is possible, however, to integrate portions of the different models into a useful approach to effective leading in programs and projects. Leading effectiveness results from interactions among variables including leader traits and behaviors selected to fit situations, all of which are mediated or influenced by intervening variables such as participants' efforts and abilities, organization design features, and the availability of appropriate inputs or resources in a program or project's logic model. Furthermore, in health programs and projects, participative styles of leading work best most of the time.

Above all else, it is important for managers to realize that because leading is a matter of influencing participants to contribute to achieving the desired results established for a program or project, they must help participants be motivated to make their contributions. Motivation is a means to the end of leading participants to contributions that help accomplish a program or project's desired results.

In terms of using motivation in the leading activity, the simplest, and perhaps best advice is to select motivated participants to fill the positions in an organization design. People who have demonstrated appropriate levels of performance in the past are motivated to perform and will quite likely continue to perform well under favorable conditions. Leading such participants to contribute to accomplishing a program or project's desired results is rather straightforward. This aside, however, some of the most significant challenges of leading and helping participants be motivated in the workplace arise because managers do not clearly define and specify the desired results (outputs, outcomes, and impact) toward which they want participants to contribute. Being an effective leader, and using motivation to support the leading activity , begins with clear statements of desired results. These statements are especially useful when those who will be influenced by them have participated in their formulation and agree with them.

The models of how motivation occurs show the powerful and direct connections among participants' efforts, performance, and rewards. A critical step in motivating people is choosing appropriate ways to reward desired performance, remembering that rewards can be intrinsically derived from the work itself, or extrinsically provided by managers.

It is also important to remember that people have different valences or preferences about rewards. Reward selection is made more difficult because of individual tastes and preferences regarding rewards. Some people would rather have more challenging assignments or more vacation time than more money. For others, the reverse is true. The point for managers to remember is that rewards must be important to the people receiving them if they are to be effective motivators. Often, valences can be determined simply by discussing the matter of their preferences with participants. Viewed broadly, their responsibilities to provide suitable rewards can lead managers into areas such as job redesign and job enrichment, changes in their leading styles, changes in the degree to which they permit others to participate in decisions, as well as concerns about pay levels and benefits.

Selecting rewards that are suitable is only part of the process of using rewards to motivate. Managers must link rewards to suitable job performance; that is, rewards must be made contingent upon performance, and the linkage must be explicit. The more a person is told about the relationship between performance (with clearly established expectations about performance) and rewards, the more likely the rewards will help motivate desired performance.

The performance-reward linkage is strengthened by having rewards follow as soon as possible after desirable performance and by providing extensive feedback on performance to participants. Finally, it is important to remember that people have a strong preference for being treated fairly or equitably. Their perceptions about the linkage between performance and rewards at work are fundamental to their sense of fairness. Managers must pay careful attention to the equity implications of their use of rewards.

We have also seen that motivation alone does not fully account for participants' performance or for their contributions to accomplishing the desired results established for a program or project. A participant's performance is also determined, in part, by the person's abilities and by constraints in the work situation such as uncoordinated workflow or inadequate budgets for technology or training. This means it is important for managers to remove or minimize barriers to performance. Barriers of inability to perform can be addressed through increased education and training and, in some cases, by more careful matching of people with positions. Situational constraints, such as inadequate inputs/resources or organization designs that impede performance, can be addressed once they are identified as constraints.

Managers' capacities to lead effectively, including using motivation to support leading, are greatly enhanced in work situations in which there is concern for the overall quality of work life (QWL). Programs and projects, and the larger organizations in which they may be embedded, can approach QWL from several specific dimensions or foci of attention, including the following:

- Adequate and fair compensation
- A safe and healthful work environment
- A commitment to the full development of participants
- A social environment that fosters personal identity, freedom from prejudice, and a sense of community
- Careful attention to the rights of personal privacy, dissent, and due process
- A work role that minimizes infringement on personal leisure and family needs
- Commitment to socially responsible organizational actions (Bateman and Zeithaml 1993)

Summary

In leading, managers of programs and projects seek to influence other participants to understand and agree about what needs to be done to achieve the desired results established for their programs or projects and to facilitate both individual and collective contributions to achieve the desired results. To lead effectively, managers must help create and maintain conditions under which other participants in a program or project can and do contribute to accomplishing the desired results established for it. Thus, an understanding of human motivation and application of the process through which motivation occurs is necessary for success in leading.

Motivation is defined as an internal drive within an individual, which is a stimulus to behaviors intended to satisfy an unsatisfied need being felt by the individual. Thus, motivation stimulates goal-directed behavior. The basic process of motivation is modeled in Figure 4.1. Overviews of the primary content and process perspectives of motivation are presented (see Figure 4.2).

Models within the content perspective focus on the internal needs and desires that initiate, sustain, and eventually terminate behavior. They focus on what motivates people. Four content models of motivation are presented: Maslow's hierarchy of needs theory, Alderfer's ERG theory, Herzberg's two-factor theory, and McClelland's learned needs theory. Process models seek to explain how behavior is initiated, sustained, and terminated. Three process models of motivation are also presented: Vroom's expectancy model, Adams's equity model, and Locke's goal-setting theory.

Motivation is a means to an end, leading participants to make contributions that help accomplish the desired results established for a program or project in terms of outputs, outcomes, and impact. However, there is more to leading than motivating participants. The evolution of leadership models is described in this chapter (see Figure 4.5).

Models of leading based on leader traits, including intelligence, personality, and ability, are reviewed. Pioneering research about leader behavior conducted at Ohio State University and the University of Michigan is presented as a prelude to reviewing the behavioral models of leading developed by Likert, by Blake and McCanse, and by Tannenbaum and Schmidt. It is noted that the Tannenbaum and Schmidt model represented a significant advance in understanding leading by recognizing that no single style of leading works best all of the time or in all situations.

Three key situational or contingency models of leading are reviewed: Fiedler's contingency model, Hershey and Blanchard's situational model, and the House-Mitchell path-goal theory of leading. How these models build on and complement one another, as well as how they differ, is described. Particular emphasis is given to contemporary situational concepts of leading.

Chapter Review Questions

1. Define leading and discuss its relationship to management work.
2. Define motivation and model the basic motivation process.
3. Compare the content models of motivation developed by Maslow, Alderfer, Herzberg, and McClelland.
4. Compare the process models of motivation developed by Vroom, Adams, and Locke.
5. Describe the relationship between influence and leading and between interpersonal power and influence.
6. Describe the sources of interpersonal power available to managers in health programs and projects and give an example of each.
7. Discuss the evolution of approaches to understanding leading effectiveness.
8. Why is the Tannenbaum and Schmidt model especially important to an understanding of leading?

CHAPTER FIVE

MAKING GOOD MANAGEMENT DECISIONS

This chapter focuses on *decision making* as a pervasive activity in management work. Managers of health programs and projects constantly make decisions while performing management work. Decision making permeates the core activities of strategizing, designing, and leading. It is a vital facilitative activity that supports managers in carrying out their core activities. Figure 1.4 shows how decision making is intertwined with the core management activities.

Examples of the decisions managers make in each of the core activities of their work illustrate the breadth of their decision-making activity. In *strategizing* the future, managers, often with the involvement of other participants, decide what will be the program or project's desired results, expressed in terms of outputs, outcomes, and impact. They also decide the means through which these desired results can and will be achieved. When managers establish new programs or projects, they must make decisions about what goes into the business plans. Numerous decisions must be made about how to conduct external and internal situational analyses. Managers make decisions about whether acceptable progress is being made toward achieving the desired future states they have envisioned for their programs and projects.

In the *designing* activity, managers make myriad decisions as they establish the initial logic models of their programs and projects and subsequently reshape them as circumstances change. They must decide what inputs/resources are needed, and how to acquire needed resources. They must decide what processes will be used to achieve the desired results established through strategizing. Other decisions are required when managers establish the intentional patterns of relationships among human and other resources within their programs and projects as they shape organization designs. The designs then stimulate other decisions regarding staffing.

In *leading,* managers must decide how to encourage and facilitate the contributions of other participants in a program or project to make its logic model work. Managers decide what means of influencing other participants will work effectively and how they will be applied. As leaders, managers focus on the various decisions that affect the entire undertaking, including those intended to ensure the program or project's survival and overall well-being. Because leading effectively requires managers to help motivate participants to contribute to the program or project's performance, they must decide how to motivate participants, each with a unique set of needs that can be met partially in the workplace.

Indeed, how managers conduct their decision making has a great deal to do with success in all the core activities of strategizing, designing, and leading. After reading the chapter, the reader should be able to do the following:

- Define decision making and understand some of the important characteristics of management decisions in programs and projects
- Understand and model the sequential steps in the decision-making process
- Be familiar with some of the most popular quantitative models that support decision making, including decision grids, payoff tables, decision trees, and cost-benefit analysis
- Understand the implementation and evaluation of management decisions as important steps in the decision-making process

Decision Making Defined

At its most basic level, decision making is simply making a choice between two or more alternatives. Thinking of decision making in this way focuses attention on its essential element—making a choice. The myriad decisions that program and project managers face can be divided into two subsets: problem-solving decisions and opportunistic decisions (DuBrin 2003). Both types of decisions involve choosing from among alternatives.

As the name implies, *problem-solving decisions* are made in order to solve existing or anticipated problems. *Opportunistic decisions* can be made when opportunities to advance accomplishment of a program or project's desired results arise, often by changing some element—perhaps a very small element—in a logic model or organization design. Examples of such decisions include an opportunity to purchase some needed equipment or supplies at favorable prices or an opportunity to recruit an especially skilled clinician for a program or project. The line is thin at times between problem solving and opportunistic decisions, but managers make both types of decisions in their work.

All management decisions are the responsibility of managers. However, managers can choose to involve to varying degrees other participants in the decision-making process. Managers can make decisions themselves, or, as is far more often the case, they can involve other participants in their programs or projects in making decisions. The question of who makes decisions in programs and projects is an important aspect of making good management decisions.

Involving Other Participants in Decision Making

Much of the literature on how managers make decisions describes the process as one in which decisions are made as relatively discrete events by managers or by managers working with others in an orderly, rational manner. In reality, decision making is more likely to be characterized by disorder and emotionality than order and rationality (Yukl 2002). This is certainly the case when groups make decisions, as is often the case in larger programs and projects.

An important model that incorporates consideration of involving other participants in decision making was developed by Vroom (1973), extended by Vroom and Yetton (1973), and subsequently revised by Vroom and Jago (1988). In this model, the approach managers take to involving other participants in decision making is shown to affect the resulting decisions in two important ways. First, the approach taken affects the quality of the decisions made. Second, the approach taken affects how people who will implement decisions or who will be affected by them will respond to the decisions. Both quality and acceptability have obvious implications for the effectiveness of decisions.

As originally developed, the Vroom model features a decision tree and a set of questions to guide users. The model assumes that managers can take any of five different approaches to including other participants in decision making. The approaches are defined and labeled as follows:

- Two types of *autocratic* decision making (AI and AII)
- Two types of *consultative* decision making (CI and CII)
- One approach that represents joint decision making by managers and other participants as a *group* (GII)

Each of these five decision-making approaches is briefly described as follows:

AI	Managers make decisions alone, using information available to them at the time.
AII	Managers obtain the necessary information from other participants and then decide for themselves. The role played by other participants is merely to provide information to managers. Other participants play no part in generating or assessing alternatives in the decision-making process.
CI	Managers share information about the problem or opportunity requiring a decision with other relevant participants individually, obtaining their ideas and suggestions, but without bringing the participants together as a group. Then managers make the decisions, which may or may not reflect the influence of the other participants.
CII	Managers share information about the problem or opportunity requiring a decision with other relevant participants as a group, obtaining their collective ideas and suggestions. Then the managers make the decisions, which may or may not reflect the influence of the other participants.
GII	Managers share information about the problem or opportunity requiring a decision with other relevant participants as a group. There is a GI approach; however it is not relevant to this discussion. In the GII approach, managers and the other participants involved generate and assess alternatives and attempt to reach agreement (consensus) on an alternative. The manager's role in this approach is much like that of the chairperson of a committee. Managers do not try to influence the group to adopt their preferred alternative and are willing to accept and implement solutions that the groups prefer.

Figure 5.1 shows the Vroom decision tree, which a manager can work through from left to right by answering seven questions (A through G in Figure 5.1) in order to conclude which of the five decision-making approaches (AI, AII, CI, CII, or GII) is most appropriate in a given situation. The questions, which correspond to the letters A through G, are shown across the top of the flowchart.

FIGURE 5.1. VROOM'S DECISION PROCESS FLOWCHART.

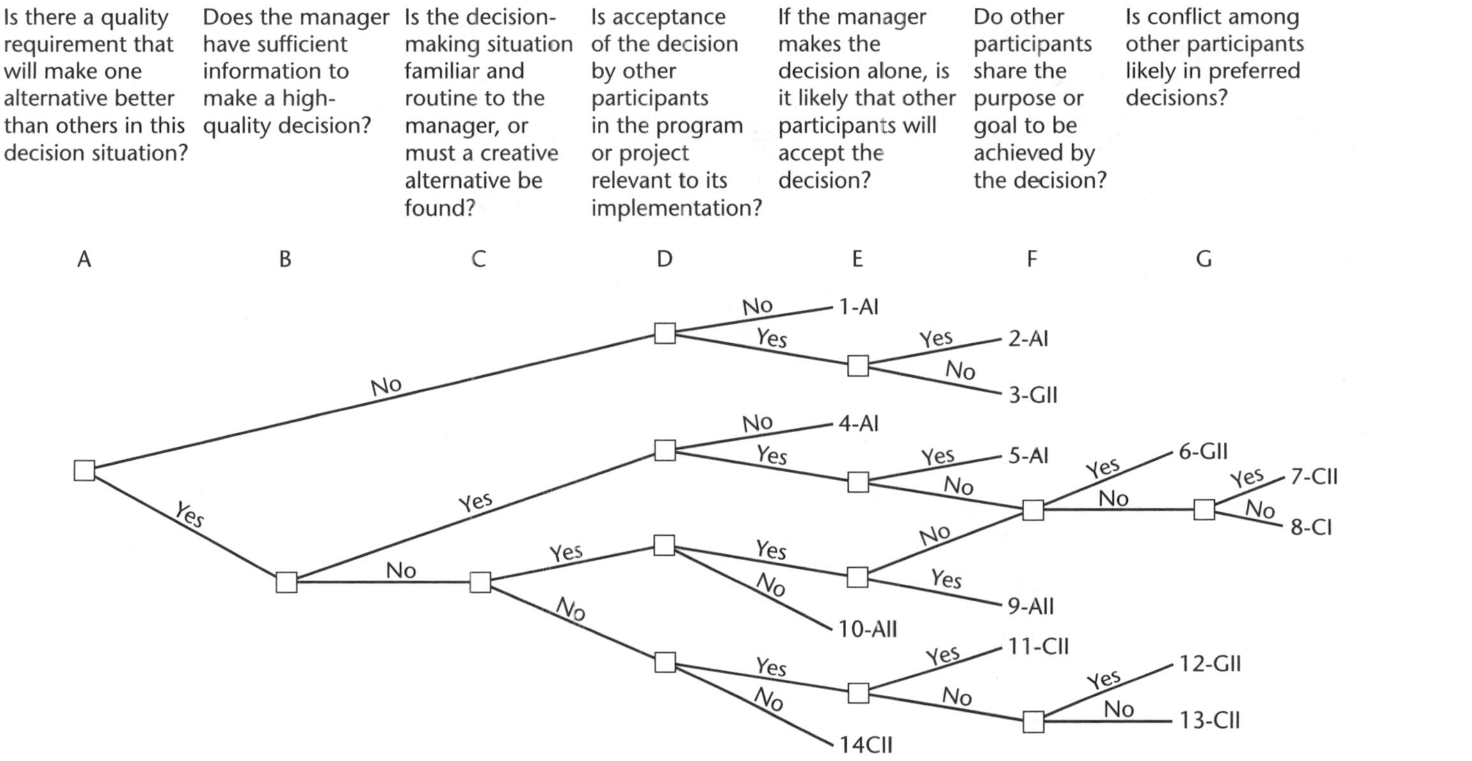

A
Is there a quality requirement that will make one alternative better than others in this decision situation?

B
Does the manager have sufficient information to make a high-quality decision?

C
Is the decision-making situation familiar and routine to the manager, or must a creative alternative be found?

D
Is acceptance of the decision by other participants in the program or project relevant to its implementation?

E
If the manager makes the decision alone, is it likely that other participants will accept the decision?

F
Do other participants share the purpose or goal to be achieved by the decision?

G
Is conflict among other participants likely in preferred decisions?

1-AI
2-AI
3-GII
4-AI
5-AI
6-GII
7-CII
8-CI
9-AII
10-AII
11-CII
12-GII
13-CII
14CII

By answering the questions in the sequence A–G, the manager reaches endpoints 1–14, each representing an autocratic, consultative, or group approach to decision making of the form AI, AII, CI, CII, or GII that is appropriate to a particular decision-making situation.

Source: Adapted from *Organizational Dynamics,* vol. 1, no. 4, Victor Vroom, "A New Look at Managerial Decision Making," pp. 66–80, copyright 1973, with permission from Elsevier.

The Vroom model has practical value for managers because it demonstrates they can effectively vary their approach to involving other participants in decision-making situations to fit attributes of the particular situation. When managers do seek the involvement of other participants as a group in decision-making situations, they can facilitate participation in several ways (Yukl 2002), including the following:

- Encouraging participants to express their ideas about alternatives in a decision-making situation and to express their concerns about other ideas being suggested
- Describing alternatives as tentative and encouraging participants to try to improve them
- Recording ideas and suggestions as a way of demonstrating their importance and that they are not being ignored
- Looking for ways to build on ideas and suggestions by focusing on their positive attributes rather than their negative attributes
- Being tactful in expressing concerns about ideas and suggestions and encouraging other participants to be tactful in how they express their concerns
- Listening to dissenting views or criticisms without getting defensive
- Actively seeking to use ideas and suggestions and to address concerns being expressed
- Demonstrating appreciation for the ideas and suggestions of other participants, especially giving credit to those who generate useful ideas and suggestions and explaining why other ideas and suggestions are not included in the decision

Even when managers correctly determine the appropriate degree of involvement in decision making by other participants in a program or project, many other variables affect the decision-making process. For example, some decisions made by managers must be based on imperfect information about available alternatives and their consequences and implications. Managers' decisions frequently involve risk, uncertainty, and conflict. These characteristics of management decisions and decision making, as described more fully in the next section, complicate the process of making such decisions, making decision making one of managers' most challenging activities.

Characteristics of Management Decisions in Programs and Projects

One of the most important and troubling aspects of making good management decisions is that they often cannot be made in a completely rational manner. The underlying assumptions for making completely rational decisions would require that decision makers know all the alternatives available in a given situation, all of the consequences of selecting each alternative, and that the decision maker would always act rationally so as to maximize a desired value or minimize an undesired value. Because it is not possible to meet all of the assumptions required of complete rationality in most management decisions, managers make decisions using a more limited form of rationality called *bounded rationality* (Simon 1982).

The assumptions of bounded rationality are that managers rarely have enough information and knowledge to maximize or minimize anything in their decision making, face vaguely defined problems or opportunities about which decisions are to be made, and have human limitations of memory, reasoning power, and objectivity. These bounds on rationality mean that managers are forced to *satisfice*. That is, in their decision making managers typically choose alternatives that appear adequate and acceptable, rather than selecting alternatives that would completely maximize or minimize some variable. The satisficer considers possible alternatives until a satisfactory one is found. Satisficing is a fact of life in making management decisions.

Another characteristic of decision making by managers in programs and projects is that decisions must often be made under conditions of uncertainty. Their decisions require managers to accept some degree of risk. Risk exists because managers cannot know with certainty the probability of success for their decisions.

Under conditions of certainty, a manager would fully understand the problem or opportunity requiring a decision, would know all of the available alternative choices, and would accurately predict the results of selecting each alternative. Managers almost never make decisions under conditions of certainty. Just as managers are forced to rely upon bounded rationality and are not able to make perfectly rational decisions, managers also typically must make their decisions under conditions of uncertainty.

Uncertainty in making managerial decisions exists because the decision makers have insufficient information about the probabilities of success for the alternatives in decision situations. Uncertainty can be reduced by the acquisition of more information, but in complex situations it cannot be completely removed. Sometimes managers are required to make intuitive decisions that are based on nothing more than instincts, feelings, and personal experience with similar situations. In contrast to decisions that can be guided by large amounts of relevant information, intuitive decisions tend to involve high degrees of uncertainty and risk.

Another important characteristic of managerial decisions is that they are often influenced by significant conflicting demands and expectations. The appropriate decision, from the standpoint of what contributes most to achieving the desired results established for a program or project, might have painful consequences for some participants. Decisions to downsize a program or to merge a project into a larger set of projects are examples of such decisions. Most managers faced with decisions such as these feel significant amounts of internal conflict.

In addition to personal conflict for the decision maker, many decisions generate conflicts between or among individuals or groups within a program or project, or even within the larger organizational home in which it is embedded. Decisions to emphasize one of a program's services automatically de-emphasize others. Decisions to allocate space to one group involved in a project automatically mean that others could not use that space. Indeed, most managerial decisions involve some degree of conflict and this makes them more difficult to make.

Situations in which management decisions are made can be characterized as structured or unstructured. Unstructured decision making occurs when problems or opportunities demand decisions but there are no existing models or formulae to call upon for guidance. This is in contrast to structured decisions, for which previously made decisions, operating policies, or standard practices provide guidance. For example, the amount of money paid to a new employee is structured by human resources policies that dictate pay ranges and by salaries paid to others with similar qualifications.

Many decisions made in the context of managing programs or projects are made difficult by such factors as the need to rely on bounded rationality and by varying levels of uncertainty, risk, conflict, and structure in the decision-making process. Some decisions that managers must make are made extraordinarily difficult by these characteristics.

The Decision-Making Process

Although decision making is defined as making a choice from among alternatives, the full decision-making process includes several sequential steps that precede the actual choice. Once the choice is made, the full process includes additional steps to implement and evaluate the decision. In reality, managers rarely go through all the steps in sequence. Frequently, under constant pressure to make decisions, managers skip or combine steps. However, as Figure 5.2 illustrates, decision makers can go through a process that includes the following seven steps:

1. Becoming aware that a decision must be made, whether it stems from a problem or an opportunity
2. Defining in as much detail as possible the problem or opportunity
3. Developing relevant alternatives
4. Assessing the alternatives
5. Choosing from among the alternatives

6. Implementing the decision
7. Evaluating the decision and making necessary follow-up decisions

Each of these steps is described in the following sections.

Becoming Aware

Effective decision makers must be sensitive to situations in their programs or projects that represent problems or opportunities. This sensitivity, termed *perceptual skill,* enables managers to collect and interpret cues from their surroundings. Managers with limited perceptual skills may remain oblivious to potential problems until they blossom into full-blown crises, or until they discover too late that they did not seize a potential opportunity. It is difficult to learn perceptual skills except through experience. Such skills are one of the reasons that managers usually become more effective with experience.

FIGURE 5.2. THE DECISION-MAKING PROCESS.

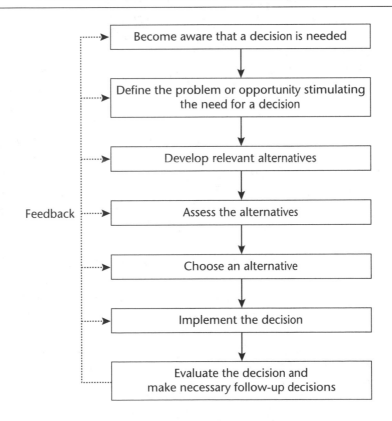

One way for managers to increase the likelihood that they will be aware of problem-solving and opportunistic situations requiring decisions is to acknowledge their ubiquity. Many decisions are required simply to respond to performance gaps in programs and projects that are routinely identified through managers' efforts to determine whether ongoing performance is acceptable and whether appropriate progress is being made toward achievement of the desired results. Remember from the discussion in Chapter Two that a key part of the manager's strategizing activity is to assess performance and progress in an ongoing manner. Managers must also make adjustments and corrections if inadequacies are detected; that is, they must change some aspect of the program or project's logic model. All such changes require decisions.

In addition to the decisions managers must make in response to closing ongoing performance gaps in their programs or projects, other decisions are imposed on them from outside their domains of responsibility. In some instances, pressure comes from inside the organizational home of the program or project. For example, a decision to merge one hospital with another, when both operate hospice programs, will necessitate many decisions in both programs.

The changes that continuously occur in the dynamic external environments in which most health programs and projects exist force decisions within the programs and projects. For example, growing, declining, or aging populations in their market areas, as well as the plans and actions of competitors, have significant implications for health programs and projects. Such environmental changes trigger numerous decisions by the affected programs and projects as their managers seek to adapt and adjust the programs and projects to fit new environmental conditions.

Changes in public policies and regulations that apply to a program or project frequently give rise to decision making. For example, changes in Medicare or Medicaid reimbursement policy routinely force decision making in health programs and projects that serve the clients of these programs. Similarly, National Labor Relations Board (NLRB) rulings can instantly change how programs or projects relate to unionized employees, again forcing decisions. Because health programs and projects so often depend on particular technologies, advances in these technologies provide a stimulus for change in the programs and projects. For example, telemedicine programs have evolved as changes in the technologies upon which they are based have occurred, with each step in the evolution requiring decisions about how adjustments to new technologies will be made.

Perceptive managers in complex and dynamic environments should be aware of the constant need for problem solving, as well as for making opportunistic decisions. Knowing that decisions are needed and knowing how to precisely define the problem or opportunity are two different things, however. This leads to the second step in the decision-making process described in Figure 5.2.

Defining the Problem or Opportunity

Defining the real problem or opportunity in a given situation is not always a clear-cut task. What appears to be the problem may be only a symptom. For example, an apparent problem of conflicting personalities when two participants in a program or project cannot work together well might in fact be only a symptom of such real problems as poorly coordinated work, conflicting scheduling, inadequate training, or ill-defined work expectations. Few things are more frustrating in decision making than the right solution to the wrong problem, unless it is the effort wasted in responding to a perceived opportunity that does not really exist.

A simple but effective way of getting past the symptom to the underlying problem or opportunity is to ask "Why?" Answers to this question can be used to trace back from symptoms to underlying root causes. Similarly, answers to questions about why some event, trend, or situation appears to be an opportunity for a program or project can also lead to a clearer specification of the opportunity.

A device useful in getting to the root causes of a problem is a *cause-and-effect diagram,* or, as it is frequently called because of its shape, a *fishbone diagram.* Figure 5.3 is a fishbone diagram drawn by the manager of a specialized surgical program embedded in an acute care hospital. The problem concerning this manager is a higher-than-expected rate of nosocomial pneumonia among patients in the program. In a fishbone diagram, the high rate of pneumonia is the effect. The manager is interested in what is causing the effect, because the cause or causes must be addressed through decisions and subsequent actions. Before this can be done, however, the manager must understand the possible causes. The issues that require decisions by this manager are the underlying root causes of the nosocomial pneumonia.

In using a fishbone diagram to organize ideas about what might be causing the nosocomial pneumonia among the program's patients, the manager begins by identifying categories of possible causes. Common causes of nosocomial infections include equipment, interventions or procedures, workers, and patients. The manager organizes the diagram around these potential categories of causes, which form the larger bones in the diagram. Within each category, specific ideas about the causes can be developed and are shown as the smaller bones in the diagram. The diagram does not identify the causes; however, it *organizes* the manager's thinking, and perhaps ideas of other participants involved in making this determination about the possible causes of high rates of nosocomial pneumonia. More information will be needed to determine the causes of the nosocomial pneumonia, but the possible causes are identified in the fishbone diagram, which is the first step in determining causation.

FIGURE 5.3. A FISHBONE DIAGRAM OF POSSIBLE CAUSES OF NOSOCOMIAL PNEUMONIA.

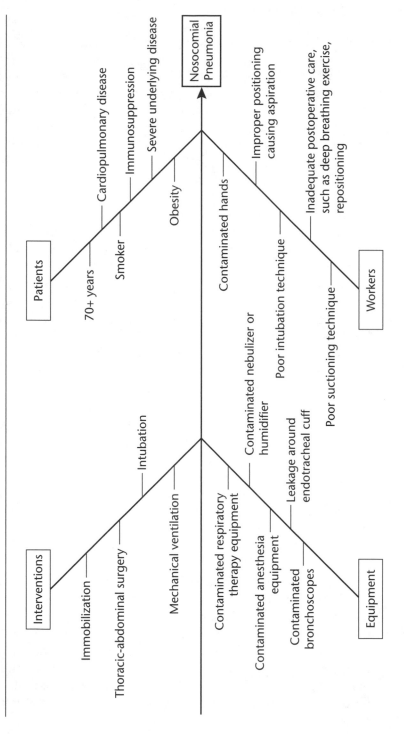

Another tool useful for this manager's determination of the causes of the pneumonia is a *Pareto chart,* a bar graph showing the relative importance of several causes of a problem. Such charts or graphs can help managers determine which causes are more important and thus where to focus their attention. Figure 5.4 is a Pareto chart showing the relative importance of the several causes of nosocomial pneumonia identified in this example; it directs the manager's attention to the most important causes that require decisions.

As can be seen in the Pareto chart, the largest number of cases of nosocomial pneumonia in the analysis is caused by contaminated bronchoscopes. The next largest number of cases is caused by patients having severe underlying disease. Inadequate postoperative care and patients with cardiopulmonary disease are tied for the third largest number of cases. Based on the information assembled in the Pareto chart, the manager would focus initial problem-solving efforts on contaminated bronchoscopes and inadequate postoperative care, variables the manager can influence. Unless the program's patient mix changes, the manager cannot do anything about some patients' underlying disease or about some patients' cardiopulmonary disease with associated higher rates of pneumonia.

FIGURE 5.4. PARETO CHART OF POSSIBLE CAUSES OF NOSOCOMIAL PNEUMONIA.

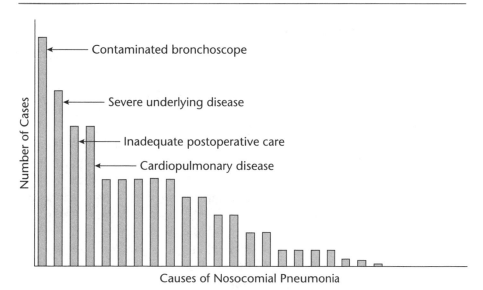

To completely diagnose problems or define opportunities, decision makers analyze a great deal of information. Judgment is required to determine what information should be used in decision making, and care must be exercised to be as comprehensive, fair, and objective as possible in gathering and examining information. The most difficult pieces of information to deal with are often intangible factors that can play a significant role in defining problems and opportunities. Intangible factors include such things as reputation, morale, satisfaction, and personal biases. It is difficult to be as specific about these subjective factors as those more easily subject to physical measurement. Nevertheless, such information must be considered in fully defining problems or opportunities.

Defining problems or opportunities is much easier when they fall within the scope of a manager's experiences. Problems and opportunities that look familiar are easier to diagnose and understand. As with being better at the awareness step in decision making, experience sharpens a manager's ability to define and specify problems or opportunities.

The degree of success in the definition step in the decision-making process is almost always directly proportional to the amount and quality of the relevant information gathered and analyzed in relation to a problem or an opportunity. Of course, good judgment is required in determining whether enough information is in hand to make an accurate diagnosis of a problem or opportunity. Generally, more information is better, but some decision makers paralyze themselves by continuing to gather information about a problem or opportunity long after they should have moved on to the next step in the decision-making process.

Developing Relevant Alternatives

Once problems or opportunities that require decisions are fully diagnosed and understood, decision makers can search for and develop alternatives. One simple rule should guide the decision maker in this step: the greater the number of alternatives considered, the greater the likelihood of eventually selecting a satisfactory alternative. Alternatives can be categorized as ready-made or custom-made.

Ready-made alternatives are based on approaches or solutions that the decision maker has tried before or on recommendations of others who have faced similar problems or opportunities. Custom-made alternatives are designed specifically for a particular decision-making situation. They generally involve greater expenditure of time and effort to develop and thus are less likely to be considered than the familiar ready-made alternatives.

In considering alternatives, decision makers should not think in terms of one best alternative. Most problems have several solutions that have both positive and negative characteristics, and many opportunities can be appropriately responded to along a continuum of possible responses. The task in developing relevant alternatives is to develop as many potentially satisfactory alternatives as is reasonably possible.

It is during this step in the decision-making process that creative and innovative alternatives can be developed if the decision maker is not inappropriately wedded to the idea of considering only ready-made alternatives. Some decision makers focus on ready-made alternatives because they doubt their abilities to develop truly creative custom-made alternatives. Creativity is the "art and science of generating new ideas" (Rice 2003, p. 22).

Logic and experience play important roles in idea generation, as does imagination. The use of imagination and creative thinking in this step of the process is important if the fullest possible set of relevant alternatives is to be established. It is useful to remember that creativity is latent within all people. Ordinary people working in an atmosphere of freedom, trust, and security can create new alternatives to problems and opportunities. Therefore it is important for managers to encourage and facilitate the use of the creative process, which is described in the next section.

The Creative Process. Embedded within the decision-making process, the creative process itself can be viewed as a series of interconnected steps, including: (1) personal need, (2) preparation, (3) incubation, and (4) verification. A personal need to think creatively emphasizes that a motivating force must initiate the creative thought process. Such motivation can certainly come in the form of a serious problem or a rich opportunity requiring a manager to make a decision.

Creative, custom-made alternatives usually emerge after a period of intensive preparation during which the decision maker becomes saturated with information and makes a concerted effort to perceive new and meaningful relationships among factors in a situation. To a large extent, the originality of ideas depends upon the number of avenues explored and the extent to which all possible interrelationships are considered. This preparatory step represents much of the work of engaging in the creative process.

It is certainly possible for an original alternative to be developed quickly as the result of a brief period of analysis. Sometimes this is necessary when an urgent decision, for which there is no ready-made alternative, is required. For example, a manager whose program faces termination may have to respond quickly and creatively if the program is to be preserved. However, when circumstances permit, a period of incubation that allows a decision maker to mull over the problem or opportunity is valuable.

The value of an incubation period lies in the fact that a more fully developed idea for a custom-made alternative may result. It is useful to set a deadline for the incubation period so that problems do not go unsolved for unduly long periods or opportunities pass while the decision maker mulls over various alternatives. But generally some period of incubation is necessary for original alternatives to be developed.

The final step in the creative-thinking process is verification. When a custom-made alternative is first envisioned, it is rarely in polished and final form. The verification step in the creative process is a period of refining an idea, changing it, and improving it. In effect, this step often represents the difference between an interesting idea and a truly innovative and creative alternative.

Sometimes the creative process is facilitated by having a group of program or project participants develop relevant alternatives in a decision-making situation. Groups of people usually bring more experience and information to the task than individuals acting alone and therefore provide more ideas for alternatives. A group, through its interactions, can stimulate each individual's creative abilities as well. *Brainstorming* is a standard method used by groups to develop alternatives in decision situations. In brainstorming sessions, participants are asked to produce ideas (without fear of censorship or control by the group), through free association of their ideas with those of others. In this way, one idea can stimulate a chain reaction of additional ideas.

Another approach to having groups establish alternatives in a decision-making situation is the *nominal group technique,* in which participants are asked to generate ideas independently (Delbecq, Van de Ven, and Gustafson 1986). Participants, working alone initially, develop their ideas. Unlike the free association of brainstorming, ideas are discussed within the group only after ideas are independently developed and presented by each participant. Following a round of discussion, during which initial ideas can be reworked, each participant privately rates the alternatives from first to last. The tabulated rankings of the group are then openly discussed again, after which a final private ranking is made. The tabulated results of this vote are considered the group's ranking of the alternatives. Both brainstorming and use of the nominal group technique result in a set of alternatives that must be assessed by the decision maker before an alternative is chosen.

Stimulating and Supporting Creativity in Decision Making. Managers who want their programs or projects to benefit from the development of creative and innovative alternatives in decision making must stimulate and support creativity and innovation. These characteristics among participants can be fostered by managers who make it a specific and important aspect of managing their programs or projects and who establish and maintain a culture in which creativity and innovation are valued. Managers can also facilitate these characteristics by placing a high priority on the trait of creativity in at least some of their staffing decisions. In effect, managers will increase the likelihood that their programs and projects will have the advantage of a more complete set of alternatives available in decision-making situations by establishing and maintaining climates in which creativity and innovation are stimulated and facilitated. Such climates share a number of characteristics (Robbins and Coulter 2004), including the following:

- Risk-taking is tolerated, even encouraged. Participants are encouraged to take risks, and mistakes are treated as learning opportunities.
- Rules, procedures, policies, and similar formally imposed controls are kept to a minimum.
- Cross-training and participation in diverse and multiple teams and groups is encouraged. Managers recognize that narrowly defined jobs create myopia, while diverse job activities and experiences give participants a broader perspective.
- Tolerance for ambiguity is widespread in the program or project. Participants are given opportunities to express their identities through work as individuals and as members of teams and groups.
- A healthy degree of conflict is permitted. Differences in opinions about how to do things is tolerated, even encouraged, as a means to increase creativity. Harmony and agreement between or among individuals and teams and groups is not seen as necessary to good performance.
- There is a high degree of tolerance for the impractical. Participants who offer improbable or even foolish answers to *what if* questions are not penalized or ridiculed. There is recognition of and appreciation for the fact that what seems impractical at first might turn out to be a great alternative in a decision situation.
- The focus is on the ends more than on the means to the ends. If participants are encouraged to consider alternative routes toward the attainment of desired results in the form of outputs, outcomes, and impact, innovation might result.
- Communication flows freely. Communication flows horizontally as well as vertically, facilitating the cross-fertilization of ideas.

Managers who wish to stimulate creativity and innovation should avoid, minimize, or change certain characteristics and behaviors. Chances of developing innovations and creative ideas are often reduced when a manager is isolated from the other participants in a program or project, when a manager focuses on short time horizons and short-term performance, and when a manager maintains incentive and reward systems that do not support innovation.

Managers who successfully rely upon their own insights and experiences, the insights and experiences of others, and the creative processes available to them will develop a set of alternatives to consider. The existence of various alternatives in a change situation requires that the alternatives be assessed against each other.

Assessing the Alternatives

Based upon the results of the creative process and the experience and insight of the manager and others, there will likely be alternatives to consider. The existence of multiple alternatives in a decision-making situation requires that each alternative be assessed in comparison to the others.

In the assessing alternatives step in the decision-making process, quantitative models can be very helpful in structuring a careful comparison of the alternatives. Five useful quantitative decision-making techniques that are widely used include: decision grid, payoff table, decision tree, cost-benefit analysis, and program evaluation and review technique. In addition, the use of decision support systems (DSSs), which combine many decision-making models with a database to support decision making, is discussed. Other quantitative techniques for managerial decisions can be found in Austin and Boxerman (1995).

Decision Grid. The most basic, and in many ways most useful, decision-making tool is the decision grid. This is nothing more than a display of the possible alternatives in a decision, along with the various elements that will affect the decision. Figure 5.5 illustrates a decision grid involving a program's decision to open and operate a satellite clinic. The four alternatives are listed in the first column, with the elements affecting the decision forming the rest of the grid. The grid's main advantage is that a large amount of pertinent information can be displayed in a convenient manner. This becomes especially important in complex decisions and when a group of program or project participants is involved in the decision making and needs to discuss and consider various alternatives.

Among the factors affecting the decision, the preferences of the program's participants is mixed for all alternatives. This neutralizes the impact of this factor. Patients/customers have a preference for alternative four, although they find any alternative acceptable except maintaining the status quo. The key factor in this decision is the financial impact of the alternative selected. Alternative four is most attractive because the financial impact is positive and almost immediate, and none of the other factors in the decision prevent selecting this alternative.

Payoff Table. An improvement in the decision grid is made if probabilities can be determined for the various possible outcomes of each alternative being assessed in a decision situation. For example, suppose the manager of a clinical

FIGURE 5.5. DECISION GRID FOR POSSIBLE ADDITION OF SATELLITE CLINIC IN A PROGRAM.

Alternatives	Patient/Customer Preferences	Program Participants' Preferences	Financial Impact	Relative Feasibility	Decision
1. Maintain status quo	Unacceptable	Mixed	Negative	Feasible, but undesirable	Not recommended
2. Purchase new site for clinic	Acceptable	Mixed	Positive over a 5-year period	Feasible, but expensive	Not recommended
3. Lease new site for clinic	Acceptable	Mixed	Positive in 2–3 years	Readily feasible	Second priority
4. Enter into an agreement to utilize a community-based organization's existing facilities for the clinic, rent-free for 10 years	Highly acceptable	Mixed	Positive within first year of operation	Highly feasible	First priority

program must decide how many disposable syringes should be ordered and stocked each week.

Based on past usage patterns, the manager determines there is an 80 percent probability that 800 syringes will be needed and a 20 percent probability that 1,000 syringes will be needed in a week. The manager can also assign costs to each of these two alternatives. In this case, storage space is allocated at $10 per 1,000 syringes. In addition, if too few syringes are ordered and stocked, an extra cost of $20 will result for special ordering and messenger pickup. Figure 5.6 illustrates the two alternatives (1,000 and 800 syringes) and the costs associated with each of the two outcomes.

For the first alternative, if 800 syringes are stocked and the usage during the week is 800, the costs will be $8 (see cell 1). If 800 syringes are stocked and 1,000 are needed that week, the costs will be $28 ($8 for storage and $20 for the special order [see cell 2]). For the second alternative, if 1,000 syringes are stocked and the usage during the week is 800, the costs will be $10 (see cell 3). Also, if 1,000 syringes are ordered and stocked and 1,000 are used, the costs will be $10.

If the clinic manager orders and stocks 800 syringes, then 80 percent of the time this decision will be correct and only an $8 storage cost will be incurred; 20 percent of the time there will not be enough and the $28 storage and reorder costs will be incurred. Expected costs can be determined for each alternative as follows:

Expected cost if 800 syringes are ordered: $8(0.8) + $28(0.2) = $12

Expected cost if 1,000 syringes are ordered: $10(0.8) + $10(0.2) = $10

FIGURE 5.6. PAYOFF TABLE.

Events and Results

		800 syringes needed (0.8)	1,000 syringes needed (0.2)
Alternatives	800 syringes stocked	1 $8.00	2 $28.00
	1,000 syringes stocked	3 $10.00	4 $10.00

Thus, to minimize costs, 1,000 syringes would be ordered and stocked, although this number would be needed only 20 percent of the time.

Although the savings is modest, if the technique is applied to many items, the cumulative savings could be quite substantial. The basic difficulty in using this technique is in determining probabilities. When possible, the preferred procedure is to use historical data or experimental samples so that the probabilities have a clear basis in fact. Where this is not possible, a best estimate may have to suffice.

Decision Tree. Decision grids and payoff tables are useful tools in assessing alternatives in a decision situation, although both suffer from a common limitation. In reality, decisions are seldom one-time affairs. They are more often linked to other decisions in the sense that one decision necessitates other decisions. In situations involving decisions that are linked together over time with various possible outcomes, decision trees are very useful in assessing alternatives. This technique is especially useful when probabilities can be determined for the possible outcomes.

To illustrate the decision tree technique, suppose the manager in a program or project determines there is a 60 percent probability that demand for a certain procedure will increase by 20 percent next year and a 40 percent probability that demand for the procedure will decrease by 10 percent. The decision is whether to buy a piece of automated equipment (at a cost of $50,000) or to pay existing employees overtime wages to do the increased work, should that be necessary. (The manager determined that it would cost less to pay overtime than to hire an additional worker.)

Because of the vital nature of the procedure, simply deciding not to do the increased work is not acceptable. Figure 5.7 illustrates a decision tree based on this decision. The decision tree assumes that quality is not an issue because it will be the same whether the procedure is done manually or on the automated equipment. Thus, the decision hinges on making the wisest expenditure of money by choosing the lowest cost alternative.

Assume that revenue from this procedure is currently $100,000 per year. If the 60 percent probability of a 20 percent increase holds up, the revenue for the next year (and future years if everything stays the same) will increase to $120,000; if the 40 percent probability of a decrease in demand of 10 percent holds, then revenue will decrease to $90,000 in both cases (see column 3 of Figure 5.7).

The cost of the machine (installation and first year's operation included) is $50,000; the cost of overtime wages is figured at $10,000 if the increased work has to be done, and at zero dollars if it does not (see column 4). Net cash flow can be determined in all events by subtracting costs from revenues (see column 5).

FIGURE 5.7. DECISION TREE.

(1) Alternative Actions	(2) Possible Events	(3) Revenue from Procedures	(4) 1st Year Costs	(5) Net Cash Flow	(6) 1st Year Expected Value	(7) 2nd Year Costs	(8) Net Cash Flow	(9) 2nd Year Expected Value
Automate	Increased demand (.6)	$120,000	$50,000	$70,000	$42,000	$2,000	$118,000	$70,800
	Decreased demand (.4)	$90,000	$50,000	$40,000	$16,000 / $58,000	$1,500	$88,500	$35,400 / $106,200
Pay overtime	Increased demand (.6)	$120,000	$10,000	$110,000	$66,000	$10,000	$110,000	$66,000
	Decreased demand (.4)	$90,000	-0-	$90,000	$36,000 / $102,000	-0-	$90,000	$36,000 / $102,000

Decision point

The expected value at the end of the first year can be obtained in all events by multiplying net cash flow (column 5) by the probability of the event. Sixty percent chance of increase times $70,000 equals an expected value of $42,000 (see column 6). At the end of the first year the expected value of automation is $58,000 (42,000 + 16,000) and of paying the overtime is $102,000. Clearly, at that point in time the lowest cost alternative would be to forgo the machine and pay overtime. However, if the decision is projected out over additional years, this may not be the lowest cost decision.

At the end of the second year (see column 9), the expected value of the alternative to automate is greater. Although the initial $50,000 outlay must still be overcome, it will not take many years to do this. By extending the computation, the number of years can be determined. When compared to the expected useful life of the machine, this information can form the basis of a complete assessment of the alternatives in this decision situation.

Cost-Benefit Analysis. A manager deciding among alternative additions to the service mix provided in a program would be interested in how the alternatives compare in terms of financial impact. A useful tool for making relative comparisons of the impact of alternatives is to calculate the cost-benefit ratio *(Z)* of each alternative. *Z* is defined as the ratio of the financial value of benefits of an alternative to the value of the alternative's costs:

$$Z = \frac{\text{present value of benefits}}{\text{present value of costs}}$$

A decision maker can assess multiple alternatives by comparing the ratios of the benefits and costs of the alternatives. Although these ratios should be only one factor in a decision, they can assist the decision maker.

Usually, it is relatively easy to determine the financial costs of an alternative. However, in health programs and projects the value of benefits is often much more difficult to determine. What is the value of a human life? What is the value of improved health? Is it better to spend money on making older people more comfortable in their declining years, or is it better to spend the money on improving infant mortality rates?

Of course, the costs and benefits of many decisions can be determined in a straightforward way. In such cases, cost-benefit analysis is a useful tool for assessing alternatives. For example, a manager might find a cost-benefit comparison very useful in assessing a choice between two competing models of a particular piece of imaging equipment.

Model A costs $80,000 (installed) and requires a person to operate it at an annual cost of $64,000, plus $12,000 in other operating costs. The total cost for a year is $156,000. Model A will produce revenues of $185,000 per year because of its rate of operation.

Model B of this equipment will have a total cost of $175,000 but will permit revenues of $205,000 because of its superior rate of operation. Which is the better alternative, assuming they both produce equal quality results and have the same useful life expectancy and salvage value?

$$\text{Model A:} \quad Z = \frac{\$185,000}{\$156,000} = 1.186$$

$$\text{Model B:} \quad Z = \frac{\$205,000}{\$175,000} = 1.171$$

All other factors being equal, the cost-benefit ratio argues that the better alternative in this situation is to purchase Model A because of its better Z value.

Program Evaluation and Review Technique (PERT). In some operational planning situations, the assessment of alternatives involves considering the timing of activities or the best sequence for a series of actions. In such situations PERT can be very useful. The basic concept used in this technique is the network, or flow plan (Kerzner 2001). The network is composed of a series of related events and activities. *Events* are required sequential accomplishment points in the program or project. *Activities* are the time-consuming elements of the program or project that connect the various events.

For example, suppose a hospital initiates a project to establish an open-heart surgery program. A number of events and activities will have to take place, including: renovation of an existing operating room, installation of new equipment, hiring and training of an open-heart surgery team, and many others. When many events and activities are involved, PERT can be very useful in making decisions about them. One alternative in this project is to do everything in a single sequence. For example, begin by renovating the operating room. Then purchase and install equipment; then hire and train the team. The flaw in this approach is that the events and activities will be strung out for an unnecessarily long time, thus delaying the project. PERT can eliminate this flaw by giving the planner a better way to time and integrate the series of events and activities.

Figure 5.8 shows a PERT network for development of an open-heart surgery program. Events are shown as boxes in the network, and arrows connecting the events represent activities. This example illustrates the three basic characteristics of a program or project that make it amenable to the PERT approach to assessing alternative sequences of actions and events. First, it must be possible to estimate how long it will take to accomplish each activity. Second, there must be definite starting and ending points. Without them, there can be no events, which are the beginning or ending of activities. Finally, and this is the key to PERT's

FIGURE 5.8. PERT NETWORK OF PROJECT TO DEVELOP AN OPEN-HEART SURGERY PROGRAM.

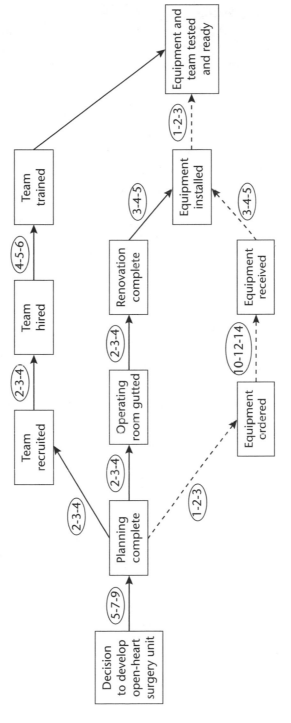

- - - - Critical path

◯ weeks Indicates, in order of listing, estimates of most optimistic, most likely, and most pessimistic completion times

usefulness, there must be parallel activities. That is, several activities must be taking place simultaneously for PERT to be of any real use to the planner.

To make the network usable, the time between the various events (activity times) must be computed. Usually, these can be only estimates, and the standard approach involves estimating three different times for each activity. The first estimate is an optimistic time and represents the time if everything goes smoothly in completing the activity. The second estimate is the most likely time and represents the most accurate forecast based on normal or typical circumstances. If only one estimate were given, this would be it. The third estimate is a pessimistic time and is based on maximum potential difficulties. The assumption here is that whatever can go wrong will go wrong. The pessimistic, most likely, and optimistic time estimates form a beta curve as illustrated in Figure 5.9.

Based on the probability distribution of the three time estimates involved in performing an activity, a formula can be used to calculate the estimated activity time to use in the PERT network as follows:

$$\text{Activity Time} = \frac{O + 4M + P}{6}$$

Where O   is the optimistic time estimate

M   is the most likely time estimate

P   is the pessimistic time estimate

Referring to Figure 5.8, it can be seen that the time estimates between the first two events have been made as follows: optimistic = 5 weeks, most likely = 7 weeks, and pessimistic = 9 weeks. The estimated activity time would then be

$$\text{Activity Time} = \frac{5 + 4\,(7) + 9}{6} = 7 \text{ weeks}$$

**FIGURE 5.9. BETA CURVE FOR OPTIMISTIC, MOST
LIKELY, AND PESSIMISTIC TIME ESTIMATES.**

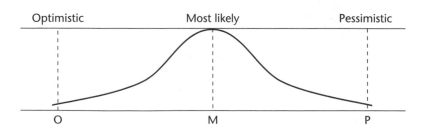

Using the resulting value, one can be reasonably certain that the activity time between events 1 and 2 will be seven weeks. The process of calculating estimated activity times must be completed for all activities in the network.

The next step in using PERT to help evaluate timing and sequencing alternatives in this example is to determine the *critical path* through the network shown in Figure 5.8. Among the several pathways of events and activities, the critical path (shown as a dashed line in Figure 5.8) is the one that takes the longest to complete. Inasmuch as the critical path takes the longest time to complete, it determines the completion time for the entire project. Other activities and events that do not lie along the critical path are less important in terms of their timing because they will not speed up or delay the total project, unless they exceed the completion time along the critical path.

The time differential between scheduled completion of these non-critical events and the amount of time that would actually alter the critical path through the project is called the *slack time* in the project. Slack time provides an opportunity for the manager to reassess whether certain resources should be transferred to activities along the critical path as a means of shortening the critical path and therefore the completion time of the project. In the example represented in Figure 5.8, it would do no good to speed up recruitment, hiring, training of the team, or renovation of the operating room in an effort to shorten the project. The only way to accomplish this is to shorten the time needed for equipment delivery and installation because these activities form the critical path in this project.

PERT, and even more sophisticated time management and scheduling techniques (Project Management Institute 2000), can be used to great advantage by managers in making timing and sequencing decisions in many building or remodeling projects, in adding new equipment, in physically moving a unit, in preparing budgets, and in developing policy manuals.

Managers of programs and projects that are embedded in larger organizations may be supported by formal planning departments and professional planners in the application of tools and aids such as PERT. Most large health care organizations employ people with such expertise in their planning, marketing, government affairs, and finance departments—and perhaps in other departments, as well. In addition, consultants can be helpful in assisting planners in assessing alternatives.

Decision Support Systems. The intensified pressure to make good management decisions in health programs and projects, combined with improved technology specifically designed to support the management decision-making process, may cause managers to consider using *decision support systems.* These systems can be defined as "computer-based technology that aims to get the right knowledge in the right form to the right persons at the right time so they can better make decisions and make better decisions" (Holsapple and Joshi 2001, p. 40). In essence, decision support systems (DSSs) incorporate data and models for analyzing the data to support decision makers in assessing their alternatives in decision-making situations.

A DSS can be constructed in various ways, although effective systems share the following characteristics:

- Interacting with the DSS is easy.
- Retrieving and displaying data is supported by the system.
- Modeling capability is built into the system.
- The system can produce reports of the results of analyses in clear and usable form (Austin and Boxerman 2003).

Figure 5.10 shows a conceptual model of the components of an effective DSS. Each of the components is described briefly in the following paragraphs.

The *user* engages the DSS through the *user interface*. The interface may use a menu format or free-text input. Whichever is used, the key characteristic is the ability to communicate with the DSS simply and intuitively.

An effective DSS contains a *model library*. The appropriate mix of models in a specific library depends upon the requirements of decision makers who use the system. Typically, a DSS designed for use in health programs and projects contains a mix of (1) *statistical models* (to summarize data, test hypotheses, make forecasts, and the like); (2) *financial models* (to predict cash flows, expenses, and revenues, as well as perform break-even analyses or compute internal rates of return on investments that might be made in a program or project); and (3) *"what if" models* that can be used to determine the effect of variation in one or more variables on a value of interest.

The *model manager* is software that links a DSS user's request to the appropriate model in the model library so the desired analysis can be conducted. The models in an effective DSS can support decision making in clinical areas (such as patient scheduling and quality assessment) as well as in non-clinical areas (such as personnel scheduling, inventory control, and accounting).

A critical part of any DSS is the *database* from which the models can draw necessary information for analysis. Depending upon circumstances in a particular situation, a program or project's database could contain data from many sources, including a clinical repository, a financial database, data developed through special studies, and even external commercially available databases. Among the specific elements that might be found in a program or project DSS database are units of service provided, resources used in providing the services, data for assessing the quality of the services (see a broader discussion of this in Chapter Seven), and data for evaluating results, whether in terms of outputs, outcomes, or impact. A database can contain data relating to any of the components of a program or project's logic model (see Figure 1.1).

The final components of a DSS are a *database management system* (software that retrieves data at the request of a user or makes needed data available to the model manager for use in a particular decision model) and a report writer, which provides a user with a report of the analysis. Depending upon the features of a DSS, the reports produced may show comparisons of several alternatives, the consequences of a particular choice among alternatives, or a recommended choice.

FIGURE 5.10. CONCEPTUAL MODEL OF A DECISION SUPPORT SYSTEM.

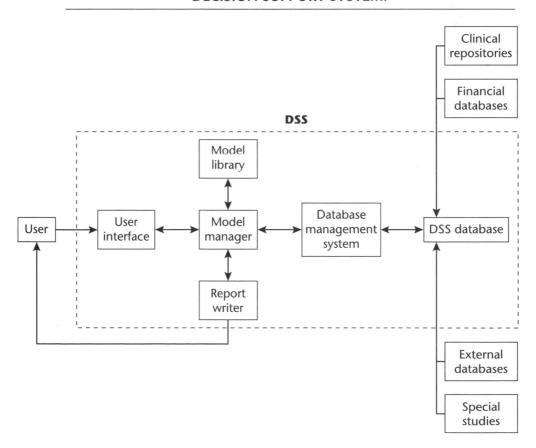

Even small DSSs costs tens of thousands of dollars and are not available to all programs and projects. However, when affordable, these systems can greatly assist decision makers in assessing the alternatives in their decision situations.

Choosing an Alternative

After developing and assessing alternatives, decision makers must choose the alternative they think best in a given decision situation. If the other steps in the decision-making process have been carried out properly, the decision maker will typically be able to choose from among several relevant alternatives.

Of course, one alternative always available is to do nothing. This should be the alternative considered most carefully of all. The decision maker should visualize the likely results of taking no action. If taking no action would result in the most desirable consequences, the decision maker should take no action. However, this alternative should never be viewed lightly. After all, a problem or opportunity—or a potential problem or opportunity—triggered the decision-making process. Unless analysis reveals there really is no problem or opportunity, the no-action alternative is usually inappropriate.

Making the choice among alternatives in a decision situation—whether based on experience, intuition, advice from others, experimentation, or analytical decision making—is rarely easy. Management decisions tend to be gray rather than black or white. They usually are made in the context of a constantly changing environment, which means that the most appropriate alternative initially may not remain the most desirable choice as circumstances change.

Aside from the difficulties encountered in collecting and properly analyzing enough information to fully inform a decision, problems can develop from the influence of the decision maker's personal prejudices and biases. These problems can interfere with a decision maker's effectiveness by forcing the selection of an alternative that fits some preconceived notion rather than the realities of a particular situation.

For some decision makers, the largest impediment to effectiveness is their own indecisiveness. On the other hand, the opposite situation can exist and may be just as detrimental to the quality of decision making. Impulsiveness, or a tendency to jump headlong into a situation without considering all factors, is not uncommon in inexperienced decision makers as they make management decisions early in their careers. If enough of their decisions turn out to be wrong, they may become indecisive. In either case the decision maker's effectiveness is diminished.

To improve the quality of their decisions, managers should answer three questions regarding the alternatives in their decision situations. First, they should ask how the alternatives contribute to the attainment of the program or project's desired results. (A discussion of development of statements of desired results is contained in Chapter Two). This question is important because it reflects the fact that the alternatives in a decision situation are but means to an end— an end that has been clearly thought out and stated in the form of outputs, outcomes, and impact. If an alternative under consideration does not support the achievement of desired results better than other alternatives, it should not be adopted.

Second, managers in decision-making situations should ask whether alternatives under consideration represent a high degree of financial effectiveness. In other words, does an alternative make maximum use of available resources? There will be times, of course, when financial considerations should not unduly affect decision making, especially in a health program or project where considerations such as need or quality may appropriately take precedence. Usually, however, financial aspects of a decision offer useful guidelines in choosing among alternatives.

Third, managers in decision-making situations should ask whether alternatives under consideration are feasible or capable of being implemented. In answering this question the decision maker must think in the very practical terms of how a particular alternative will be implemented within the context of the program or project's logic model and organization design.

Answering these three questions does not guarantee that the best alternative— or even a good one—will be chosen. Doing so, however, increases the chances for an appropriate selection.

Implementing the Decision

The process of decision making does not end with the selection of an alternative. Managers are concerned about the effects of their decisions. Thus, the implementation of decisions is an important step in the overall decision-making process. A well-chosen alternative, poorly implemented, can be useless or even harmful to a program or project. Successful implementation of a decision requires careful planning of how the implementation will take place.

Planning for Implementation. Ideally, there are three interconnected components to good planning for implementing a decision: (1) conducting a situational diagnosis, (2) selecting a general approach to implementing the decision, and (3) selecting a set of techniques to support the decision and its implementation and to reduce resistance from those affected by the decision. Each component is an important precursor to successful implementation.

The conduct of *situational diagnosis* as part of implementation planning is a natural extension of the information gathering effort that occurs in the second step of the decision-making process described earlier. During the second step, the nature of the problem or opportunity facing the decision maker is fully explored.

However, the situational diagnosis that precedes implementation of an alternative goes well beyond the information needed to identify the nature of a problem or opportunity. It includes collecting information about resources available for implementing the chosen alternative as well as information on the views and attitudes of key participants (and perhaps others outside the program or project) about the choice that has been made. It is necessary to know about resource availability and constraints before the actual implementation begins because this information can influence the selection of a general implementation strategy.

In selecting a general approach to implementation, the decision maker can choose from among three broad categories: top-down, bottom-up, or participative approaches. In *top-down approaches,* which are also called power strategies, the decision maker simply announces to other participants in a program or project the decision that is to be implemented, and explains how it is to be implemented. The other participants are expected to accept the decision and take whatever part they are told to take in its implementation.

Power approaches are necessary and appropriate in some situations. For example, a change in the reimbursement policy of a major insurance carrier might require an immediate decision in a health program or project, leaving little time for anything but a top-down edict as a means of implementing the decision(s) made in response to this problem. Top-down approaches to implementing decisions have the advantage of speed because decisions can be communicated quickly to affected participants in a program or project. On the other hand, a major drawback of top-down approaches is disruptiveness, particularly if those affected do not accept or understand the decision.

In *bottom-up approaches* to implementing decisions, participants in a program or project other than its manager have a much greater responsibility for developing details of how to implement a decision. In this general approach, the manager permits and encourages participants to decide how best to implement the chosen alternative. The primary advantage of bottom-up approaches to implementing decisions is that they foster widespread commitment to accomplishing the implementation task within a program or project.

In *participative approaches* to implementing decisions, participants responsible for implementation are involved in the entire decision-making process, along with the manager. Participation is formally sought through such devices as assigning participants to groups or teams specifically created to develop alternatives, to choose among alternatives, and to implement an appropriate alternative in response to a problem or opportunity. Participatory leading styles are discussed extensively in Chapter Four.

Implementation that involves a higher level of participation obviously differs from a top-down approach in which the decision maker's edicts announce decisions and instruct others as to how implementation of these decisions will take place. Participatory implementation approaches and strategies also differ from bottom-up approaches. Bottom-up approaches to implementation tend to focus on implementation details rather than on permitting participants to be involved more fully in the entire decision-making process, as is characteristic of true participative approaches.

The third component of good planning for implementing a decision involves *selecting techniques that help develop support for implementation and for reducing resistance* to the decision and to its implementation. In considering useful support techniques, decision makers should remember that people respond to many types of change, including that resulting from the implementation of decisions in predictable, often negative, ways. Responses are based on their prior experiences in situations in which implementing a decision includes changing some aspect of the work situation.

Although managers might view changes resulting from implementing decisions made in response to problems or opportunities as entirely appropriate and logical, other participants in programs and projects, looking at the same problems or opportunities and the changes made in response to them, might overtly resist the changes. Resistance may seem an inappropriate response to managers, but this response may seem perfectly reasonable to the resistant participants, especially if their past experiences with similar situations were negative.

One of the underlying reasons some participants view change negatively and resist it is their personal history, including their backgrounds and social experiences away from work. That is, their attitudes and reactions at work are affected by their lives outside of work. A second cause is the work environment itself. For example, if a program or project has been very stable for a long period of time, it may be especially difficult to introduce changes. Decisions that represent change for participants may therefore be resisted. When participants have adjusted to the status quo and believe it is permanent, the introduction of even minor changes can be disruptive. Conversely, in programs or projects with histories of frequent change and in which change is seen as part of the culture, participants expect change and much more readily accept it.

There are many other reasons for the often-encountered resistance to change among participants in programs and projects, including the following:

- Feelings of insecurity
- Fears of possible social and economic losses, to say nothing of actual losses
- Distaste for being inconvenienced
- Resentment that others are exerting control over them

Insecurity among affected participants is a major source of resistance to decisions that involve changes. For many people, there is great comfort in the status quo, and any change is viewed as undesirable because it introduces a degree of uncertainty. Even a seemingly simple change can have far-reaching repercussions. For example, changing the schedule of meetings for a program or project's participants may symbolize for some the manager's lack of concern for inconvenienced participants. To others, it means true interference with other aspects of their work schedules or routines. A third group may see it as more evidence of the autocracy of managers.

Participants also may be concerned about social losses of various kinds that could result from a particular decision. Even the potential of such losses can cause people to resist a particular alternative in a decision situation. For example, modifications in the organization design of a program or project may mean that close friends have to work in separate rooms or are no longer able to interact during work. Complex informal relationships among participants are often affected by change. Established status symbols may be destroyed in the process of reorganizing a program or project.

Social acceptance by other participants may be jeopardized if someone supports an alternative that these co-workers have rejected. In such circumstances, a person may be forced to choose between cooperating with the manager or jeopardizing friendships and acceptance by other participants. Thus, what may seem a desirable and logical alternative in a decision can meet with heavy resistance because the price in social relationships is too high.

Possible social losses are not the only concerns participants in a program or project may have about alternatives under consideration. Real or perceived economic losses may also be involved. In many situations new technology allows more work to be done by the same or even fewer people. Resistance by those affected is understandable. Even if they don't lose their jobs or have their earnings reduced, workers may find technological changes lead to a faster pace of work or to a redistribution of their workload. Economic losses frequently are of concern to people who face changes in their workplaces. People are therefore likely to resist decisions that create such changes.

Even when decisions do not cause significant economic or social losses, participants may be inconvenienced because of a decision. Any change causes some inconvenience, and extra effort is required to adjust to it. When old habits and routines must be replaced because of a decision, inconvenience often stimulates resistance. However, if inconvenience is the only factor present, the degree of resistance may be minor.

There are many reasons for the often-encountered resistance to particular alternatives in a decision situation. People affected by the decision may resist for reasons ranging from little more than their dislike of being inconvenienced by the decision, to concerns about a decision's economic impact on them, to such complex factors as resentment of the manager's power to affect them so directly. These and other factors cause people to resist decisions and their implementation, and the factors often act in combination to strengthen the resolve of people to resist. However, managers can use a variety of techniques to help overcome resistance.

Key to any effort to reduce resistance is informing and educating those affected by a decision about the decision and its implications *before* it is implemented. Effective communication about a change and education regarding its implications can turn resistance into support.

Participation and involvement in the entire decision-making process, including how best to implement decisions, can help overcome resistance. Such involvement reduces uncertainty and misunderstanding about a decision and its implications and reduces resistance. Participating in decisions about implementation provides an opportunity for people to gain a clearer picture of the changes that might occur as a result and enhances their commitment to successful implementation.

Facilitation and support techniques managers may find useful to help participants accept decisions include training programs, granting requests for leave during a painful transition period, or even special counseling sessions for people adversely affected by a decision. Sometimes, in exchange for participants' support of a decision, it is possible to mitigate resistance by giving additional resources or a promise to make a desired change at a later date.

Typically, the necessary set of support-enhancing and resistance-reducing techniques forms a *package* of techniques aimed at different participants whose resistance must be overcome. Selecting and packaging the appropriate set of techniques to support the implementation of a decision and reduce resistance to it, as well as selecting a suitable general approach to implementing the decision, both of which should be based on a thorough situational diagnosis, are important precursors to the successful implementation of decisions. However, planning for implementation must be followed by actual implementation.

Actual Implementation. The actual implementation of a decision involves three distinct steps: *unfreezing* the status quo, *changing* to a new state, and *refreezing* to make the new state permanent, at least until a future decision triggers a new round of implementation (Lewin 1947). Figure 5.11 illustrates the steps in the Lewin model of implementing a decision. Using the general approach selected to implement a decision, whether a top-down, bottom-up, or participative strategy, the manager or others responsible for the implementation first unfreezes the status quo. Once the status quo is unfrozen, change can occur. In a top-down approach, a simple announcement of a decision and plans for its implementation can unfreeze the status quo. A more elaborate participatory approach can also be used to unfreeze the status quo and initiate change.

FIGURE 5.11. LEWIN'S THREE STEPS IN IMPLEMENTING CHANGES.

Step 1: Unfreezing

The manager's task is unfreezing the status quo and preparing those who will participate in or be affected by a decision and the resulting change.

This is done by

- Making people aware of the decision and impending changes
- Reducing or minimizing people's resistance

Step 2: Changing

The manager's task is introducing the actual change necessitated by a decision.

This is done by

- Inserting different concepts or ideas, practices, or physical things into a situation

Step 3: Refreezing

The manager's task is refreezing the situation with the implemented decision and resulting change in place.

This is done by

- Restabilizing the situation
- Establishing conditions that will contribute to permanence

If the change is physical, such as purchase of a new piece of equipment, it is put in place and people begin using it. If the change is a concept or practice, such as new reporting relationships in a revised organization design for a program or project, a new marketing strategy, or a modified accounting system, it is initiated and people begin using it.

The third step in implementing a decision involves incorporating the changes into the routines of those carrying out the implementation. In effect, a new equilibrium is established as people adapt and accept the decision as the norm.

There is no assurance that a decision can be implemented, no matter how appropriate a response to a problem or an opportunity, or how carefully its implementation is planned. However, managers can take certain actions to increase the likelihood their decisions will be successfully implemented. Most important is for managers to be certain that participants involved in implementing a decision understand the situation fully. Participants who understand the necessity and appropriateness of a particular decision are more likely to adjust to it.

Managers implementing a decision should provide information as far in advance as possible and include specifics of the reasons for the decision, its implications, the timing of its implementation, and the expected impact on the program and project, as well as on its participants.

Some decisions can be implemented on a trial basis. When feasible, this should be considered by the manager. Familiarity gained through experience with the implementation of a decision, along with assurances that the decision is not irrevocable, can reduce initial concern and increase the likelihood of acceptance. Allowing time for assimilation of changes that result from the implementation of a decision may also increase ultimate acceptance by those involved. It is also useful when implementing decisions to minimize disturbing customs and informal relationships. Change almost invariably disrupts the culture in which it occurs. Minimizing such disturbance is facilitated by widespread participation in the entire decision-making process. Participants feel less threatened by resulting changes that they help plan because they understand them better, and they are usually more committed to the successful implementation of decisions if they are involved in the entire decision-making process.

Evaluating the Decision

The final step in the decision-making process outlined in Figure 5.2 is often given inadequate attention by managers and may be overlooked altogether. Managers must evaluate their decisions because they have a responsibility to optimally use resources entrusted to them as they manage their programs or projects. Almost all managerial decisions involve expending resources such as money and time, which have alternative uses. Systematic evaluation determines if the resources used as a consequence of decisions yield benefits such as improved or enhanced quality, efficiency, satisfaction, adaptiveness, and survival potential sufficient to justify the decisions.

In addition, evaluation provides a basis for feedback, which can lead to adjustments in previous decisions in the form of new or modified decisions. The evaluation of decisions requires collection and assessment of information and data on how well the decision is working, on whether the decision has been effectively implemented, and, most importantly, whether the problem or opportunity that triggered the decision-making process has been either solved or successfully seized.

Information showing that results do not match those intended provides feedback to the decision-making process. The manager may cycle back to the first step in the decision-making process by becoming aware that a problem or unmet opportunity still exists. The process begins again, this time with more information, new insights into what might or might not work, and a bit more experience with the challenging process of making managerial decisions in the context of programs and projects. Alternatively, as shown by the feedback loop in Figure 5.2, the cycling back can be to any prior step in the decision-making process, where adjustments can be made in the continuing effort to solve a problem or take advantage of an opportunity.

Summary

Decision making is defined as making a choice between two or more alternatives. It is critical to effectively performing the strategizing, designing, and leading activities in management work.

A seven-step process of management decision making is presented in the chapter as follows. (Figure 5.2 shows the process.)

1. Becoming aware that a decision must be made, whether stemming from a problem or an opportunity
2. Defining the problem or opportunity in as much detail as possible
3. Developing relevant alternatives
4. Assessing the alternatives
5. Choosing from among the alternatives
6. Implementing the decision
7. Evaluating the decision and making necessary follow-up decisions

Several analytical tools that can be helpful in evaluating the alternatives in a decision situation are described. Most basic is the decision grid, which displays possible alternatives in a decision situation along with the various elements that will affect each. A payoff table is more useful than the decision grid in situations where probabilities can be assigned to various possible outcomes. The decision tree illustrates the necessity, in many cases, of realizing that decisions are not one-time affairs. More often, one decision necessitates future decisions. The decision tree is a tool that can be helpful in evaluating decisions linked together over time with various possible outcomes. Cost-benefit analysis can be a useful tool, too, so long as decision makers recognize the difficulty in determining the true costs and benefits of various alternatives. The program evaluation and review technique (PERT), which can be very useful in considering the timing of activities or the best sequence for a series of actions, is discussed. The general structure of a decision support system (DSS) is presented.

Many factors enter into successful decision making by managers, including experience, intuition, advice from others, experimentation, and analysis. Effective decision makers take advantage of all these aids in carrying out their decision-making responsibilities because their decisions within programs and projects are often fraught with uncertainty, risk, and conflict.

Chapter Review Questions

1. Define decision making and describe some of the most important characteristics of management decisions.
2. List the sequential steps in the decision-making process and describe each briefly.
3. Discuss creative thinking as a component of developing alternatives in decision situations.
4. Describe some of the commonly used quantitative models available to help decision makers choose from among alternatives in decision situations. What is a DSS?
5. Discuss the three interconnected components of good planning for implementing decisions.
6. Discuss the three steps involved in implementing a decision. What can managers do to improve the chances for successful implementation?
7. Why is it important for managers to evaluate their decisions?

CHAPTER SIX

COMMUNICATING FOR UNDERSTANDING

This chapter focuses on *communicating,* a pervasive activity that is both vital to the successful performance of management work and a challenge for managers (Ross, Wenzel, and Mitlyng 2002). Communicating involves senders, who can be individuals, groups, or organizations, conveying ideas, intentions, and information to receivers, who can also be individuals, groups, or organizations. Communication is effective when receivers understand ideas, intentions, or information as senders intend.

Like decision making, communicating is a *facilitative* activity that managers engage in as they perform their core activities of strategizing, designing, and leading as depicted in Figure 1.4. When managers interact with other participants in strategizing the future of a program or project they must communicate about the desired results in terms of outputs, outcomes, and impact. They must also communicate about the means through which these desired results will be sought. When managers develop a business plan for a new program or project, they prepare a document to use in communicating their ideas to others. When managers assess whether or not acceptable progress is being made toward achieving the desired future states they envision for their programs or projects, and take corrective actions to address deficiencies in the progress, these actions depend upon effective communication.

In the designing activity, managers communicate as they develop the initial logic models of their programs and projects and when they subsequently reshape them as circumstances change. They also communicate about the implications of the logic models for participants affected by them. Further communication is required when managers establish the intentional patterns of relationships among human and other resources within their programs and projects as they shape organization designs. Still other communications are necessary as managers staff the designs.

In leading, managers communicate extensively with other participants in a program or project as they encourage and facilitate their contributions to making its logic model work. Because leading effectively requires managers to help participants be motivated to contribute to the program or project's performance, managers must communicate with participants about their needs and about how these can partially be met in the workplace.

Like making good decisions, communicating effectively greatly impacts the degree of success managers achieve in their core activities of strategizing, designing, and leading. In addition, effective communication is vital to managing quality, as will be discussed in Chapter Seven, and is crucial in marketing, as will be discussed in Chapter Eight. After reading this chapter, the reader should be able to do the following:

- Define communicating and model the basic communicating process
- Appreciate the importance of communicating effectively with internal and external stakeholders
- Understand the contextual and personal barriers to communicating effectively and how to manage these barriers
- Understand how communication flows within programs and projects and how these flows are combined into patterns called communication networks
- Understand the importance and mechanisms of informal communication
- Understand the special challenges and importance of communicating with a program or project's external stakeholders

Communicating: Key to Effective Stakeholder Relations

All programs and projects have a variety of *stakeholders,* the individuals or groups with a *stake* or significant interest in the program or project (Fottler 2002). Managers must communicate effectively with the *internal stakeholders* within their programs and projects *and* ensure effective communication between their programs and projects and a wide variety of its *external stakeholders*. Internal stakeholders are the participants in a program or project, whether employees or volunteers. External stakeholders include a program or project's existing and potential patients/customers, as well as accrediting agencies, competitors, government (as both payer and regulator), insurance plans, media, and suppliers, among many others. Figure 6.1 is an external stakeholder map for a health program. Such a map can be uniquely drawn for any program or project.

Communicating with stakeholders provides many opportunities for managers to put into practice their commitment to ethical behavior. The reader may wish to review the section on ethically managing programs and projects in Chapter One. The guidelines to ethical behavior presented in that discussion boil down to the following simplification: "Generally speaking, behaving ethically means avoiding lying, cheating, and stealing, as well as cruelty, deception, and subterfuge" (Seglin 2002, p. 76). This is useful guidance for communicating with those who have a stake in a program or project.

FIGURE 6.1. EXTERNAL STAKEHOLDER MAP FOR A HEALTH PROGRAM.

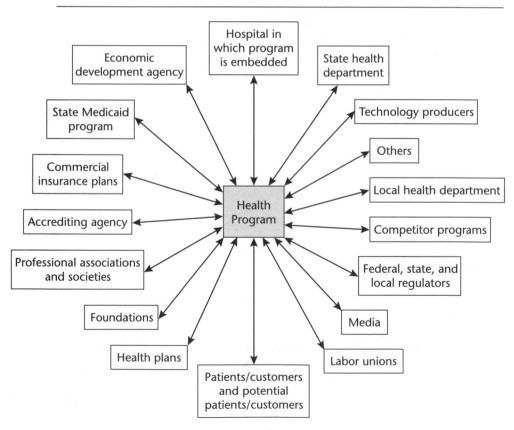

FIGURE 6.2. TYPICAL RELATIONSHIPS BETWEEN PROGRAMS OR PROJECTS AND THEIR STAKEHOLDERS

Typically *Positive* Relationships	Typically *Neutral* Relationships	Typically *Negative* Relationships
Participants	Accrediting agencies	Competitors
Patients/customers	Foundations	Regulators
Suppliers	Non-competing programs or projects	Media

Relationships with internal and external stakeholders vary along a continuum of positive to neutral to negative, with positive and negative relationships varying in intensity. Figure 6.2 represents examples of the internal and external stakeholders of programs and projects arrayed according to the typical—but by no means universal—nature of the relationships with these stakeholders. Although in Figure 6.2, stakeholders occupy *typical* patterns of relationships, patterns may vary among programs and projects. The pattern is unique for each program or project, depending upon its circumstances. It is important to note that managers can alter these relationship patterns. It is possible, for example, to move a relationship with a stakeholder from negative to neutral or positive.

Positive and neutral relationships with stakeholders provide better starting points for effective communication than do negative relationships. Therefore, managers improve their chances of communicating effectively with stakeholders by maximizing the proportion of stakeholders with whom their programs and projects enjoy positive relationships and by minimizing negative relationships. Because the intensity of positive and negative relationships varies, the manager's objective is to cultivate strongly positive relationships. Since neutral relationships are better than negative ones, but not as good as positive relationships, it is desirable to take steps to convert neutral stakeholders to positive ones.

Establishing and maintaining positive relationships with both internal and external stakeholders requires considerable sustained effort. In essence, as managers seek to establish and maintain good relationships with stakeholders they attempt to do the following:

- Achieve among internal and external stakeholders a widespread understanding and acceptance of the desired results (outputs, outcomes, and impact) established for a program or project, as well as of its logic model and organization design

- Garner support for and secure contributions toward achievement of desired results from stakeholders
- Achieve and maintain a workable balance between the program or project's desired results and the needs and preferences of its stakeholders

Relationships between programs and projects and their stakeholders can be effectively managed in two ways, both heavily dependent upon communicating effectively. A manager can seek to establish and maintain good relationships with stakeholders by fitting a program or project's logic model, organization design, and performance to the preferences, requirements, and expectations of its stakeholders. Alternatively, a manager can seek a closer match between a program or project and its stakeholders by changing the stakeholders in some way.

In trying to fit the program or project to the preferences, requirements, and expectations of its stakeholders, the manager uses knowledge of these preferences, requirements, and expectations–at least in part–to guide decisions that mold the program or project into a form that facilitates positive stakeholder relationships. The necessary knowledge about the preferences, requirements, and expectations of internal and external stakeholders is obtained by communicating with them.

Efforts to build positive internal stakeholder relationships by fitting a program or project to the preferences, requirements, and expectations of internal stakeholders are exemplified by the provision of more satisfying working conditions or by better pay and benefits for participants. An example of building positive external stakeholder relationships is responding to the identified preferences of patients/customers. For example, the provision of childcare for patients/customers while they receive services might be in response to expressed preferences for such service. Or a program or project might redesign its physical layout to appeal to and accommodate an older clientele if they understand this preference through communicating effectively. In each case, the program or project is altering or reshaping itself in some manner to better fit the preferences, requirements, and expectations of some of its external stakeholders. By doing this, stakeholder relations are likely to be improved.

In the second approach to managing stakeholder relationships, managers can seek to alter stakeholders in order to achieve a closer match between the stakeholders' preferences, requirements, and expectations and the program or project. This approach also depends upon communicating with the stakeholders.

Examples of efforts to build better relationships through changing internal stakeholders include providing additional training and education for participants to better equip them to contribute, using participative decision-making processes to gain participants' commitment to implementing decisions, and adding new participants with needed expertise to the staff. When such efforts work, the internal stakeholders better fit the needs of the program or project and the relationship is improved.

Examples of efforts intended to influence external stakeholders include marketing activities designed to educate and inform potential patients/customers about services, and communication intended to provide useful information to regulators as they consider approval of a new technology. If these communication efforts succeed, better and more positive relationships will exist between the program or project and the stakeholders.

A Model of the Communicating Process

In communicating, as was noted previously, senders, who can be individuals, groups, or organizations, convey ideas, intentions, or information to receivers, who can also be individuals, groups, or organizations. The ideas, intentions, and information are conveyed through an exchange process as depicted in Figure 6.3. When the exchange process works well, the receiver understands the idea, intention, or information. However, conveyance of ideas, intentions, or information between senders and receivers is more readily and easily accomplished than achievement of understanding.

FIGURE 6.3. A MODEL OF THE PROCESS OF COMMUNICATING.

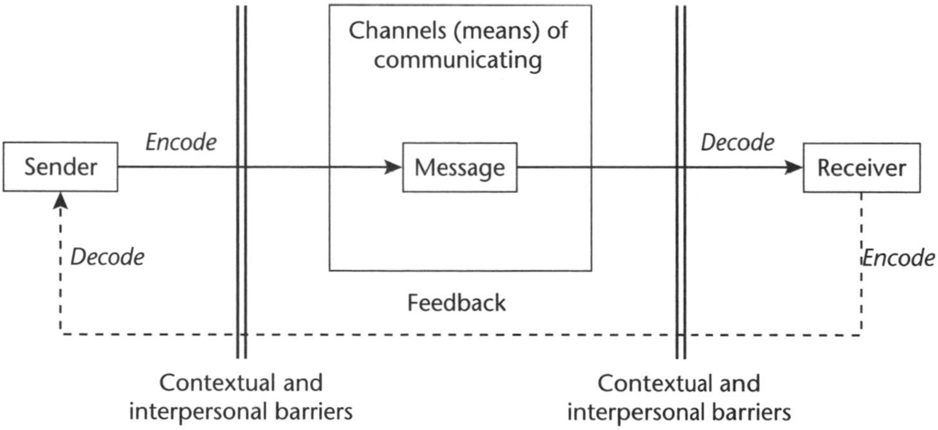

Regarding the components of the communication exchange process depicted in Figure 6.3, *senders* want *receivers* to understand their *messages*; that is, senders want their messages *decoded* exactly as they were *encoded*. Unfortunately, understanding can be difficult to achieve because of the many *contextual* and *interpersonal barriers* to effective communication. *Channels* are the mechanisms through which messages are conveyed, including face-to-face or telephone conversations, e-mail, facsimiles, letters, memoranda, policy statements, work schedules, reports, electronic message boards, teleconferences, newspapers, television and radio commercials, and newsletters for internal or external distribution.

Ideally, communication exchanges include a *feedback* loop. The chances of effective communication are improved if receivers provide feedback to senders, who can then adjust the message if it is not received as intended. When a sender encodes and transmits a message to a receiver who decodes the message and indicates understanding by giving feedback, effective two-way communication occurs.

In the model of communicating shown in Figure 6.3, senders use words and symbols to encode ideas, intentions, and information into a message for receivers. Because words can have different meanings for people, care must be taken to communicate in words that are easily understood and perhaps augmented with other symbols. Communicating is not restricted to words alone because achieving understanding may require multiple channels, including both verbal and nonverbal means. Even silence conveys meaning and is thus a means of communicating.

In health programs and projects, many symbols have a role in communication. These symbols can be physical things, pictures, or actions. For example, a particular uniform (physical thing) may permit quick identification of people in some health care settings. Everyone knows who wears the long white coats.

Pictures or visual representations are another type of symbol that can increase understanding in many situations. Consider how many words, in lieu of a chart such as Figure 3.5 or 3.6, would be needed to explain the organization design of a large program. Or, imagine the difficulty of using only words to communicate all the information in a sophisticated image of a patient's heart.

Finally, action is a symbol that communicates. A smile or a congratulatory handshake has meaning. A promotion or pay increase conveys a great deal to the recipient, as well as to others. Lack of action can also have symbolic meaning. When managers fail to follow through on promises of new resources or promotions, or fail to acknowledge work that is done especially well, they are sending clear messages.

Actions or inactions that are inconsistent with words transmit contradictory messages. The manager who tells a participant, "I have confidence in your ability; your performance is excellent, and I want to expand your duties by delegating more to you" who then becomes angry when the participant makes a small technical error is acting inconsistently. The receiver who says, "I am listening," to the sender and then looks at the clock impatiently or starts to walk away while a conversation is under way sends a mixed message.

The selection of channels is an important part of the communication process. Communicating effectively often involves using multiple channels to convey a message. For example, a major revision in the desired results established for a program or project might be announced in a letter or memorandum from the manager to all participants, graphically illustrated by posters in key locations, and then reinforced in group meetings where the manager explains the change and responds to questions about it.

A decision to lobby the state legislature for more generous Medicaid reimbursement might result in messages conveyed through channels such as letters to individual legislators, direct contact between managers and legislators, and newspaper advertisements stating the program or project's position. If others would benefit from the legislation, they might participate–perhaps through an association–in producing and distributing television commercials or using other channels to increase support for increased Medicaid funding.

Those who receive messages must decode them, no matter what channels are used in conveying the message. The surest way to determine if messages are received as intended is through feedback. In the absence of feedback, communication is a one-way process. Feedback can be direct or indirect. Direct feedback is a receiver's response to a sender regarding a specific message. Indirect feedback is more subtle, involving consequences that result from a particular message. For example, indirect feedback on a message about changing a program or project's physical location might include higher levels of participant satisfaction if the change is liked, or increased turnover among participants if the change is disliked. Similarly, indirect feedback on communication intended to change Medicaid reimbursement levels might include an increase in rates if the legislature agrees with proponents of the increase, no action if they disagree, or even hostile action if they disagree with the message and are upset by the means used to communicate.

Explicit attention to each element in the communication process shown in Figure 6.3 can improve a manager's effectiveness at communicating. For example, a sender wishing to improve communications could be concerned about how the intended receiver processes information. The sender might consider whether the receiver is better able to interpret information received verbally or in writing.

A simple way of improving communication is for senders to cue receivers as to the purpose of their messages. For example, it will help a receiver to know whether the purpose of a message is to provide information, to elicit a response or reaction, or to support a particular alternative in a decision-making situation. Communication can be improved if the sender carefully considers the content, importance, and complexity of messages in determining the channels through which the messages are communicated. Similarly, the time frames associated with particular communication situations should be considered in choosing the channels through which messages are sent. That is, faster channels and more precise cues are needed with shorter time frames. Paper memoranda are too slow to use in effectively communicating emergency situations, for example.

No matter how carefully and skillfully a manager communicates, there are almost always barriers that must be overcome if communication is to be effective. These barriers apply whether a manager is communicating with internal or external stakeholders.

Barriers to Communicating Effectively

The contextual and interpersonal barriers depicted in Figure 6.3 are ubiquitous in the communicating process for managers in health programs and projects, whether communicating with internal or external stakeholders. Contextual barriers of several types arise in programs and projects, including in the organizational homes in which many are embedded. Interpersonal barriers arise from the nature of individuals and their interaction with others as they communicate. Contextual and interpersonal barriers can block, filter, or distort messages as they are encoded and sent, or as they are decoded and received. Overcoming these barriers is vital to communicating effectively. Understanding the barriers is the first step in addressing them.

Contextual Barriers

Common contextual barriers found in programs and projects (as in all busy work settings) include competition for the attention and time of both senders and receivers. For example, multiple and simultaneous demands on a sender may cause a message to be encoded inadequately; similar demands may also interfere with its receiver causing the message to be incorrectly decoded. In such situations, a receiver may receive a message without comprehending it because the receiver is not giving the message sufficient attention. Similarly, time constraints may be a barrier to effective communication by giving a sender inadequate opportunity to think through and carefully structure a message to be conveyed, or by giving its receiver too little time to determine its meaning.

Other contextual barriers include the complexity of the organization design of a program or project and the prevailing attitude about communication that can affect senders and receivers alike. The existence of multiple levels in a program or project's design, as well as other organizational complexities such as size and diversity of activity, creates barriers that tend to cause message distortion.

As messages are transmitted up or down through a hierarchy of levels in a program or project, and as participants at each level interpret the messages according to their personal frames of reference and vantage points, there are many opportunities for information to be filtered, dropped, or added, or for emphasis to be rearranged. As a result, messages sent through many levels are more likely to be distorted. Furthermore, there are more opportunities for messages to be blocked as they are transmitted along a chain of participants. A message sent from a manager to participants through several layers of a program or project may be received in quite a different form than originally sent. Or a report prepared for the manager that passes up through layers in an organization design may not reach its destination because it is blocked along the way.

In addition to the structural aspects of a program or project that can interfere with the communication process, the attitudes about communication in a particular context can either facilitate or serve as a barrier to communicating. A manager's attitude about communication can significantly inhibit or promote effective communication. As a rule, managers who are not interested in promoting communication within a program or project will establish procedural and organizational blockages, which are serious contextual barriers to effectively communication. Symptoms of an anti-communication attitude that invariably retards communication include: requiring all communications to flow through formal channels; being inaccessible; showing a lack of interest in participants' frustrations, complaints, or feelings; and not allotting sufficient time to communicate.

Managers' attitudes about communicating also significantly impact communications with external stakeholders. Differences in attitudes could lead two managers to act very differently in communicating with external stakeholders in a crisis. For example, knowledge that patients/customers might have been exposed to a dangerous infection while being served in a program could lead one manager to conceal this information, whereas another manager faced with the same situation would make wide use of the public media hoping that everyone who might have been exposed would come forth to be tested and treated as needed. These different reactions would reflect, in part, different attitudes about the role of communicating in management work.

A final contextual barrier that may cause a breakdown in communication lies in the messages themselves. When messages contain specific terminology unfamiliar to the receiver or when messages are especially complex these features can be barriers. Each profession has its own jargon. Managers of programs or projects may use very different terminology (terms such as *payoff tables* or *logic models,* for example) than terms used by participants who are responsible for direct or support work. Routinely, many of the participants in health programs and projects use terminology that is unfamiliar to external stakeholders.

Communication between people who use different terminology can be ineffective simply because people attribute different meanings to the same words. When a message is both complex and contains terminology that is unfamiliar to the receiver, it is especially likely that misunderstanding will occur. This contextual barrier is widespread in communicating within health programs and projects as well as between them and many of their external stakeholders.

Interpersonal Barriers

Interpersonal barriers are always possible in the communicating process because the process involves people interacting with others. The interpersonal relationships that exist among participants within a program or project can promote effective communication, but they can also distort the encoding or decoding of messages, or inhibit their conveyance. For example, a discordant relationship between a manager and another participant in a program or project can dampen the flow and content of information between them and can certainly interfere with achieving understanding.

In some instances, a participant's past experiences may inhibit communicating because of fear of reprisal, negative sanctions, or ridicule. For example, it is not unusual to find participants in programs and projects who are reluctant to communicate with managers because of negative past experiences when communicating that something was wrong or when disagreeing with a manager's idea or decision. On the other hand, good interpersonal relationships, especially those characterized by trust, generally support and facilitate communication.

When people encode and send messages or decode and receive messages, they tend to do so according to their personal frames of reference. They also may consciously or unconsciously engage in selective perception, or be influenced by fear or jealousy in communicating.

Socioeconomic backgrounds and previous experiences largely determine individuals' frames of reference, which shape how messages are encoded and decoded, or even whether communication is attempted. For example, someone whose cultural background emphasizes not challenging authority may be inhibited in communicating with organizational superiors. Naive people tend to accept communication at face value without filtering out erroneous information or noticing gaps in the information they receive. Self-aggrandizing people may send distorted messages intended to provide them some advantage or gain for themselves.

Furthermore, unless all those involved in communication exchanges have had similar experiences it may be difficult to completely understand the messages they exchange. The wealthy may have difficulty understanding the concerns of people without health insurance. Those who have never experienced serious illness or loss of a loved one may be unable to fully understand messages about these experiences.

Closely related to the different frames of reference of individuals are their differing values and prejudices, which can cause messages to be distorted in sending or receiving. They can also cause messages to be blocked. Different values and prejudices are apparent in people around issues such as politics, ethics, religion, fairness in the workplace, race, and lifestyle. Their differing values and prejudices filter and distort communication and therefore impede effective communication.

Selective perception is another interpersonal barrier. People often screen derogatory information and amplify words, actions, and meanings that flatter them; people tend to filter out the "bad" of a message and retain the "good." Selective perception can be conscious or unconscious. When it is conscious, often because one fears the consequences of the truth, intentional distortion results. For example, managers whose programs or projects have high rates of turnover among participants may fear that those they report to will notice it. They might argue that turnover is due to low wages over which they have no control (or responsibility), or delete, alter, or minimize the importance of this information in reports to their organizational superiors.

Sometimes jealousy, especially when coupled with selective perception, may result in conscious efforts to filter and distort incoming information, transmit misinformation, or both. For example, a manager with a superb assistant who routinely makes the manager look good may block or distort information that would reveal this fact to organizational superiors, preferring that they give the manager full credit. Sometimes nothing more than petty personality differences, the feeling of professional incompetence or inferiority, or greed can lead to jealousy and result in communication distortion.

Another potential interpersonal barrier to communicating effectively arises because people receiving messages have a tendency to evaluate and judge the sender. Receivers often evaluate the source of a message in order to decide whether to filter out or discount part of the message. Participants who distrust a manager, for example, may ignore messages from the manager; or managers may ignore messages from program or project participants with whom they frequently disagree. Source evaluation may help communicators cope with the barrage of messages exchanged in typical health programs and projects, but it also can mean that legitimate messages are misunderstood.

A final interpersonal barrier to effective communication is a lack of empathy on the part of communicators. Having empathy means being sensitive to the frames of reference or emotional states of other people in the communicating situation. Such sensitivity promotes understanding. Empathy helps the sender decide how to encode a message for maximum understanding and it helps the receiver interpret the message's meaning. For example, participants in a program or project who empathize with its manager may discount an angry message because they are aware that extreme pressure and frustration is causing such a message to be sent even though it is not warranted.

Similarly, a sender who is sensitive to the receiver's circumstance may decide how best to encode a message or decide that it is better left unsent. For example, if a participant is having a bad day, a reprimand may be interpreted more negatively than intended. If a participant has just emerged from a traumatic experience such as family illness, the empathetic manager might decide to delay bad news until later. A manager who is empathetic with external stakeholders might delay announcing a generous across-the-board wage increase or a substantial price increase just after a major local employer announces a plant closing in the community.

Minimizing Barriers to Communicating Effectively

Awareness that contextual and interpersonal barriers to effective communication exist is the first step in minimizing their impact. However, overt actions are needed to overcome them. Although the specific steps necessary to overcome the barriers depend on circumstances, several general guidelines can be suggested.

Contextual barriers are reduced if a culture is established within a program or project that encourages and facilitates communicating. These barriers can also be reduced if receivers and senders ensure that attention is given to their messages and that adequate time is devoted to sending and receiving messages.

Reducing the number of links (levels in the hierarchy of a program or project's organization design, or steps between a program or project as a sender and its external stakeholders as receivers) through which messages pass reduces opportunities for distortion. For example, a flat organization design may mean that a message from a program or project manager can go to all participants simultaneously rather than moving through two or three levels in a tall organization design. Similarly, an e-mail message sent directly to an external stakeholder rather than a letter that passes through one or more assistants before being read by the intended receiver may enhance understanding. Consciously tailoring words and symbols so messages are understandable and reinforcing words with actions significantly improve communication among people with different positions. Finally, using multiple channels to reinforce complex messages decreases the likelihood of misunderstanding. For example, a message sent through e-mail, followed by discussion of the issue in staff meetings, and reinforced with an explanatory memorandum including background data uses three channels to reinforce the message and to minimize misunderstanding.

Interpersonal barriers to effective communication are reduced by conscious efforts of sender and receiver to understand each other's frame of reference. Recognizing that people engage in selective perception and are prone to jealousy and fear is a first step toward eliminating, or at least diminishing, these barriers. Empathy with those to whom messages are directed is one of the surest ways to increase the likelihood that the messages will be received and understood as intended.

Both contextual and interpersonal barriers can be overcome or minimized by effective *listening* within the communication process. Rice (2003) suggests the following good listening habits:

- Clear away physical distractions such as noise or interruptions.
- Express your interest in listening.
- Maintain your focus while listening.
- Ask questions as you listen.
- Listen with your mind as well as your ears.
- Take notes whether you need to or not.
- Listen early and often.

Communicating Within Programs and Projects

Communications flow downward, upward, horizontally, and diagonally within programs and projects. Each direction has its appropriate uses and unique characteristics (see Figure 6.4). Typically, downward or upward flow is communication between organizational superiors and subordinates in a program or project; this flow is typical of communication between managers and other participants. Horizontal flow is between organizational equals such as between managers of similar sections or subunits of a program or project, or between co-workers. Diagonal flow cuts across sections or subunits and levels.

FIGURE 6.4. COMMUNICATION FLOWS IN
PROGRAMS AND PROJECTS.

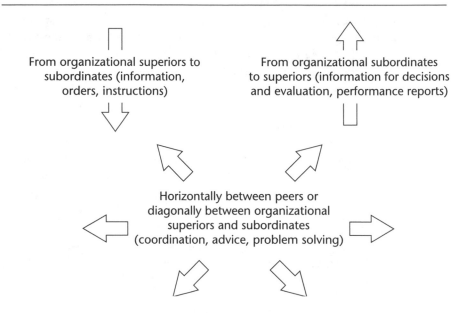

From organizational superiors to subordinates (information, orders, instructions)

From organizational subordinates to superiors (information for decisions and evaluation, performance reports)

Horizontally between peers or diagonally between organizational superiors and subordinates (coordination, advice, problem solving)

Downward Flow

Downward communication primarily involves transmitting information from organizational superiors to subordinates. It commonly consists of information, verbal orders, or instructions from organizational superiors to subordinates transmitted on a one-to-one basis. It also may include speeches to groups of participants in meetings. The myriad written means of communicating through handbooks, procedure manuals, newsletters, bulletin boards, and memoranda also are channels of downward communication. Computerized information systems contribute greatly to downward flow in many contemporary health programs and projects.

Upward Flow

Upward communication primarily involves providing managers with information to be used in decision making, revealing problem areas, providing data for performance evaluation, indicating the status of morale, and in general underscoring the thinking of the manager's organizational subordinates. Upward flow becomes more important with increasing size and complexity in the organization design of a program or project. Managers rely on effective upward communication and they encourage it by creating a climate of trust and respect as integral components of their program or project's culture.

In addition to being directly useful to managers, upward communication flow helps other participants in a program or project fulfill personal needs. It permits them to feel a greater sense of participation and typically increases their level of satisfaction in the work setting. The hierarchical chain of command is the main channel for upward communication in most organizations, including programs and projects. However, upward communications may be supported with grievance procedures, open-door policies, counseling, questionnaires and surveys of participants, exit interviews, and participative decision-making techniques.

Horizontal and Diagonal Flows

No matter how smoothly downward and upward communication flows in a program or project, especially in one that is subject to abrupt demands for action and reaction, horizontal flow also must occur. For example, when the work of interdependent components of a program or project must be coordinated, horizontal flows of communication are necessary.

Diagonal communication flows can also be vital in a program or project. For example, diagonal communication is necessary if a program's pharmacist is to alert a physician about a potential adverse reaction between two medications ordered for a patient. Diagonal flows violate the usual pattern of upward and downward communication flows by cutting across a program or project's sections or subunits, and these flows violate the usual pattern of horizontal communication because the communicators are at different hierarchical levels. Yet, such communication is vital in many health programs and projects.

In addition to diagonal flows that result when individuals take the initiative to communicate in this way, committees, groups, or teams made up of participants from different levels of a program or project can serve as useful mechanisms of diagonal communication. In fact, the prevalence of committees, groups, and teams in health programs and projects is largely attributable to a need for horizontal and diagonal communication flows.

Grouping permits participants from different components of a program or project, including those from different hierarchical levels, to overcome many of the contextual or personal barriers to effective communication as they discuss and clarify issues and common concerns, identify potential problems, solve problems face-to-face, and coordinate activities. However, it is important to remember that groups have negative potential as well. As a group develops cohesion and commitment to common purposes, attitudes and norms within the group can facilitate or impede group performance. Group decision making can be time

consuming and expensive and a group's decisions often are compromises. For-
tunately, there is abundant guidance available in the literature on developing effective groups by taking advantage of their positive potential while avoiding
the negative (Hackman 2002; Harris and Sherblom 2002).

Communication Networks

Downward, upward, horizontal, and diagonal communication flows can be combined into patterns called *communication networks*. The networks are formed when
channels connect communicators. Three common communication networks–
chain, wheel, and all-channel–are illustrated in Figure 6.5. The *chain network* is
the standard pattern for communicating upward and downward between organization superior and subordinate pairs of participants involved in a program or
project. An example is a program in which a staff nurse (organization subordinate) reports to a nurse manager (organization superior of the staff nurse and
organization subordinate of the program or project director), who reports to
the program or project director (organization superior of both the staff nurse
and the nurse manager).

The *wheel pattern* shows a situation where eight organizational subordinates
report to one superior. This pattern can be expanded to include any number of
subordinates reporting to a superior. For example, two social workers in a project can report to a single superior, as can a larger number of social workers. The
all-channel network permits each communicator in a network to interact with every
other communicator in the network.

FIGURE 6.5. COMMON COMMUNICATION NETWORKS IN PROGRAMS AND PROJECTS.

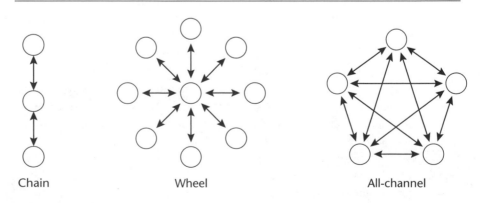

Chain   Wheel   All-channel

Communication networks vary along several dimensions and none is best in all situations. The wheel and all-channel networks tend to be fast and accurate compared with the chain network, but the chain pattern promotes clear-cut lines of authority and responsibility. The all-channel network enhances morale among those in the network because everyone is equal in the communication activity; the drawback is that communication is relatively slow. Slow communication is a serious problem if an immediate decision is needed or if an action must be taken quickly. Managers should choose networks to fit the various communication situations they face.

Informal Communication

Coexisting with the formal communication flows and networks that are established as part of the organization designs of health programs and projects are *informal communication flows,* which have their own networks. Informal flows and networks result from the interpersonal relationships among participants. Informal communication flows are often referred to as the *grapevine,* a term that arose during the early war-time use of telegraph lines strung between trees much like a grapevine. A communicator wishing to give credence to a rumor could claim that it came over the grapevine.

By definition the grapevine, or informal flow of communication, consists of channels that result from the interpersonal relationships among participants in programs and projects. Informal communication flows are as natural as the patterns of social interaction that develop in all work situations. The reader may wish to review the discussion of informal aspects of organization designs in Chapter Three because, just as informal designs coexist with formal designs, informal communication flows coexist with the formal patterns established by managers. There is no doubt that informal communication channels can be and routinely are misused in health programs and projects, especially in transmitting rumors. Yet, properly managed informal communication flows can be useful.

Downward flows move through the grapevine much faster than through formal channels. In many programs and projects, much of the coordination among clusters of work groups occurs through informal give and take in informal horizontal and diagonal flows. In the case of upward flow, informal communication can be a rich source of information about performance, ideas, feelings, and attitudes. Because of its potential usefulness and its pervasiveness, managers should try to understand informal communication flows and use them to advantage.

Similar in concept to formal communication flows, informal flows also follow certain predictable patterns and form identifiable networks. One pattern resembles a string in which participant A tells participant B, who tells C, who then tells D, and so on, until twenty participants later, Y gets the information—late and inaccurate.

A more typical pattern for informal communication flows follows a pattern in which participant A tells several others (C, D, and F). Only one or two of these receivers pass the information forward, and they usually tell several other participants. As the information grows older and the proportion of those knowing it gets larger, spreading gradually ceases. This network is a cluster chain, because each link in the chain tends to inform a cluster of other people instead of only one person as in the string pattern.

Informal communication flow is present in every health program and project and can either aid or inhibit managers in their efforts to attain suitable levels of desired results. Managers can use this flow to advantage by paying close attention to it (even inaccurate rumors may reflect certain aspects of participants' feelings and views) and by occasionally and selectively using the informal communication flow, especially when speed is critical.

To summarize, each of the communication flows and the networks they form within programs and projects serve a purpose. To the extent these flows are planned and designed by managers, they are part of a program or project's formal organization design and they represent formal communication channels and networks. To the extent they result from the natural communication between and among people arising outside the formal design, they are informal communication channels and networks. Understandable messages, whether they flow through formal channels or flow through the informal give and take among participants, are as crucial to the life of a health program or project as the circulation of blood is to human life.

Communicating with External Stakeholders

In addition to communication that occurs within health programs and projects, managers also communicate extensively with their programs and projects' external stakeholders. As noted earlier, these stakeholders include the people a program or project serves (such as its current and potential patients/customers), as well as others (such as those depicted in the stakeholder map in Figure 6.1). Effective communication between a program or project and each of its external stakeholders is necessary because the programs or projects are affected, sometimes quite dramatically, by what external stakeholders think or do.

Boundary spanning is another name for the process through which managers of health programs and projects communicate with external stakeholders.

Although managers of programs or projects that are embedded in larger organizational homes may have help with boundary spanning efforts, they are the primary *boundary spanners* for their programs or projects.

On the one hand, as boundary spanners, managers obtain information from external stakeholders that can be useful to their programs or projects. Obtaining demographic information about a service area for use in strategizing about a program or project's future service mix is an example of this sort of boundary spanning. Obtaining information about possible changes in an important regulation affecting a program or project is another example.

On the other hand, boundary spanners also represent their programs or projects to their external stakeholders. Examples of this include activities undertaken in marketing or through public relations, patient/customer relations, government relations, or community relations. Because information is the object of boundary-spanning activities–whether obtaining information from the external stakeholders or providing information to them about the program or project– communicating is critical to successful boundary spanning. Gleaning useful information from external stakeholders or effectively representing a program or project to stakeholders requires effective communication.

The technical process of communicating with external stakeholders is no different than the process used within a program or project, as depicted in Figure 6.3. Furthermore, as is the case with communication flows occurring within programs and projects, contextual and interpersonal barriers to effective communication affect communications that flow between a program or project and its external stakeholders. However, some aspects of communicating with external stakeholders deserve additional attention.

Receiving Messages from External Stakeholders

Being a good receiver when communicating with external stakeholders requires a systematic approach. Although approaches for systematically listening to external stakeholders vary, these efforts generally include a set of interrelated steps that are closely akin to the external situational analysis conducted by managers in their strategizing activity. (The reader may wish to review the discussion of this topic in Chapter Two.)

Managers who are interested in being good receivers of messages from their program or project's external environment begin by *scanning* to identify its important external stakeholders. *Tracking* the views, preferences, and positions of the stakeholders identified follows this step. The third step is *assessing* the implications of the stakeholders' views, preferences, and positions for the program or project. Finally, receiving messages effectively from external stakeholders involves *disseminating* the information received in the first three steps to program or project participants who need to know the information.

Scanning involves acquiring and organizing important information about a program or project's external stakeholders. This often is a matter of judgment, which can be improved by having multiple people involved in making the judgments through such mechanisms as ad hoc committees, task forces, or use of outside consultants. One output of such an effort is an external stakeholder map, a diagram that shows the program or project at the center with its various external stakeholders radiating out like the spokes of a wheel (see Figure 6.1).

Tracking or monitoring stakeholders' views, preferences, and positions on issues of relevance to the program or project is critical when views, preferences, and positions are dynamic, ambiguous, or simply poorly structured and unclear. Monitoring stakeholder views, preferences, and positions clarifies the degree to which they are, or the rate at which they are becoming, important or relevant to the program or project. As an extension of their tracking and monitoring efforts, managers will benefit from forecasts of likely changes in stakeholders' views, preferences, and positions. Accurate forecasts give managers time to factor the views, preferences, and positions of stakeholders into their decisions.

It is important for managers to scan and track the views, preferences, and positions of a program or project's external stakeholders. Accurately forecasting trends in this information adds to the information's value to managers. However, managers must assess and interpret the relevance, importance, and implications of information obtained from external stakeholders.

Finally, managers must disseminate the information to those who need it. This step is frequently undervalued in receiving information from external stakeholders and sometimes overlooked altogether. Unless relevant information is disseminated effectively, however, it does not matter how well the other steps are performed. Dissemination of important information obtained from or about a program or project's external stakeholders completes the process of receiving information from them. Given the vital linkage between programs and projects and their external stakeholders such as current and potential patients/customers, payers, and regulators, it is unlikely that any program or project can succeed without an effective process through which its managers routinely receive information from external stakeholders.

Of course, as with communicating effectively within programs or projects, communication between managers and external stakeholders flows two ways.

Programs and projects are both senders and receivers in communicating with their external stakeholders. Two of the most important types of communicating with external stakeholders occur in marketing a program or project and with contacts in the public sector, especially as managers advocate in support of their programs and projects or on behalf of patients or consumers.

Communicating in Marketing

Marketing is discussed in depth in Chapter Eight. Suffice it to say, the central purpose of marketing is to support the voluntary exchange of something of value between buyers and sellers (Kotler 2002b). Successful programs and projects produce services or products that are of value to certain people, groups, or organizations (for example individual patients/customers, health plans, or government agencies) and make the services or products available to them. In turn, individuals, groups, or organizations seek out the services or products and choose them. Communication is vital to how this process occurs; indeed communicating effectively is necessary for the exchanges to occur at all.

Marketing can assure that a program or project has patients/customers for its services or products, that their needs are identified and met, and that the program or project receives value in return (Berkowitz 1996; American Organization of Nurse Executives 1999). The major activities in commercial marketing include the following:

- Determining what groups of potential patients/customers (or markets) exist.
- Determining patients/customers' needs.
- Identifying which of these groups of potential patients/customers the program or project wishes to serve. In essence, these activities determine a program or project's target markets. If there are competitors for a program or project, it is also necessary to determine what competitors are doing or may do in regard to the target markets.
- Assessing the program or project's current service mix or product line relative to the identified target market's needs in order to determine what products or services the program or project can provide in response, or can develop and then provide.
- Deciding how to facilitate exchanges between the program or project and its target markets and implementing these decisions. Prerequisites to mutually satisfactory exchanges between a program or project and its target markets include responding to how and where customers prefer to gain access to and use the products and services, as well as developing pricing structures

that both attract patients/customers and provide the necessary financial resources to support the program or project. Accomplishing both requires communicating information effectively to the target markets.

- Carrying out all the activities involved in commercial marketing depends on information being exchanged through effective communication. Similarly, as can be seen in the discussion of the topic in Chapter Eight, effective communication is essential in the use of social marketing techniques in programs and projects.

Communicating with the Public Sector

Health programs and projects are affected by public policies such as laws and regulations. For example, some policies may determine vital reimbursement for a program or funding for a project. Other policies pertain to regulation of a program or project, regulation of technologies used by it, or licensure of the participants who work in it. There are also public policies that impact on the direct work of programs and policies. Seatbelt and motorcycle helmet laws are obviously of interest to programs and projects focused on highway safety, and laws related to smoking in public places are of interest to programs and projects focused on smoking cessation. The impact of public policies on health programs and projects makes effectively communicating with the public sector important.

Managers have two important categories of communicating responsibilities regarding the public sector. First, they are receivers of information from the public sector. They must acquire sufficient information to understand the consequences for their program or project of events and forces in the public sector. In effect, they listen to the public sector, using previously discussed techniques such as scanning, tracking, and assessing.

In addition to receiving information from the public sector, managers also send information to this sector. They do this in order to influence formulation of new policies, modification of existing policies, and implementation of policies in ways that support their programs or projects. So long as these efforts are made ethically and through appropriate means such as advocacy, managers act responsibly when they seek to help shape public policies in ways that enhance their programs or projects. As Figure 6.6 indicates, managers of programs and policies have many available avenues through which to help influence public policies.

FIGURE 6.6. INFLUENCING PUBLIC POLICY.

Managers can influence the formulation or modification of policy by doing the following:

- Helping shape the policy agenda by defining and documenting problems that need to be addressed, developing and evaluating solutions to the problems, and shaping the political circumstances affecting problems and solutions

- Helping develop specific legislation by participating in the drafting of legislation or testifying at legislative hearings

- Documenting the case for modification of policies by sharing operational experiences and formal evaluations of the impact of policies

Managers can influence the implementation of policy by doing the following:

- Providing formal comments on draft rules and regulations

- Serving on and providing input to rulemaking advisory bodies

- Interacting with policy implementers

> Exerting influence on public policy through each of the means listed previously requires effective and persuasive communication.

Source: Adapted from Longest, Beaufort B., Jr., *Health Policy in the United States.* Chicago: Health Administration Press, 2002.

Advocacy, which is defined as the effort to influence public policy through various forms of communicating persuasively, is a primary mechanism through which program and project managers can influence public policy. It has been argued that every manager involved in health services is an advocate and that success at advocacy depends directly on communicating effectively (Filerman and Persaud 2003).

Figure 6.7 illustrates advocacy as a six-step process that involves analysis, strategy, mobilization, action, evaluation, and continuity. For more information about these steps, refer to http://www.jhuccp.org/topics/advocacy.html.

FIGURE 6.7. "A" FRAME FOR ADVOCACY.

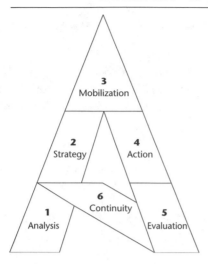

Analysis
Analysis is the first step to effective advocacy, just as it is the first step to any effective action. Activities or advocacy efforts designed to have an impact on public policy start with accurate information and in-depth understanding of the problem, the people involved, the policies, the implementation or non-implementation of those policies, the organizations, and the channels of access to influential people and decision makers. The stronger the foundation of knowledge on these elements, the more persuasive the advocacy can be.

Strategy
Every advocacy effort needs a strategy. The strategy phase builds upon the analysis phase to direct, plan, and focus on specific goals and to position the advocacy effort with clear paths to achieve those goals and objectives.

Mobilization
Coalition-building strengthens advocacy. Events, activities, messages, and materials must be designed with our objectives, audiences, partnerships, and resources clearly in mind. They should have maximum positive impact on the policy-makers and maximum participation by all coalition members, while minimizing responses from the opposition.

Action
Keeping all partners together and persisting in making the case are both essential in carrying out advocacy. Repeating the message and using the credible materials developed over and over help to keep attention and concern on the issue.

Evaluation
Advocacy efforts must be evaluated as carefully as any other communication campaign. Since advocacy often provides partial results, an advocacy team needs to measure regularly and objectively what has been accomplished and what more remains to be done. Process evaluation may be more important and more difficult than impact evaluation.

Continuity
Advocacy, like communication, is an ongoing process rather than a single policy or piece of legislation. Planning for continuity means articulating long-term goals, keeping functional coalitions together, and keeping data and arguments in tune with changing situations.

Source: Adapted with permission of the Center for Communication Programs, Johns Hopkins University, Bloomberg School of Hygiene and Public Health. (See http://www.jhuccp.org/topics/advocacy.html for more information.)

Communicating When Something Goes Wrong

Based on a large-scale study of medical errors (Brennan and others 1991), Figure 6.8 indicates the types of things that can go wrong in clinical settings. One of the verities of life for managers of health programs and projects is that on occasion, even in well-managed programs and projects, something will go wrong (Kohn, Corrigan, and Donaldson 2000). After all, many programs or projects employ, under fallible human direction, dangerous drugs, devices, and procedures in their battles against disease and injury. This is complicated by the fact that these technologies are employed on behalf of people at vulnerable stages or moments in their lives, people who often have an inflated and unrealistic expectation of what can be done for them or their loved ones.

Clinical mishaps are not the only potential problems in health programs and projects. Many programs and projects are also important economic entities in the organizations in which they are embedded, and some larger programs or projects

Figure 6.8. Types of Errors in Clinical Settings.

Diagnostic

Error or delay in diagnosis
Failure to employ indicated test
Use of outmoded tests or therapy
Failure to act on results of monitoring or testing

Treatment

Error in the performance of an operation, procedure, or test
Error in administering the treatment
Error in the dose or method of using a drug
Avoidable delay in treatment or in responding to an abnormal test
Inappropriate (not indicated) care

Preventive

Failure to provide prophylactic treatment
Inadequate monitoring of condition or progress or inadequate follow-up
treatment

Other

Failure of communication
Equipment failure
Other system failure

Source: Adapted with permission from Leape, Lucian L., Ann G. Lawthers, Troyen A. Brennan, and William G. Johnson, "Preventing Medical Injury," *Quality Review Bulletin,* Vol. 19, No. 5 (May 1993): 144–149.

even play important economic roles in their communities. Programs or projects employ people, buy goods and services, and generate costs for others who pay for their services. The finances and operations of programs and projects provide another set of things that can possibly go wrong. Financial problems in health programs and projects not only affect internal stakeholders, but also may have ramifications for external stakeholders. Indeed, health programs and projects provide ripe conditions for things to go wrong and for there to be serious consequences when they do. It is on such untoward occasions that managers' actions may matter the most.

There are direct and indirect consequences when something goes wrong in a health program or project. Clinical mistakes can cause pain and suffering directly, even death. Downsizing, laying participants off, or even terminating a program or project due to funding shortages is obviously felt directly by those who work in affected programs or projects, but may also ripple out into surrounding communities.

There are also important indirect consequences when things go wrong. Health programs and projects often are integral components of habitable, stable communities. People want networks of supportive institutions in their communities. In addition to valuing jobs and economic security, people tend to value good schools, comforting centers of religious life, responsive governments, effective public safety systems, and accessible, high-quality health services. Anything that diminishes these vital signs of stability and well-being also diminishes the quality of life. If something goes seriously wrong in a visible health program or project, it will invariably have a disturbing effect on its internal and external stakeholders and intensify the need for effective communication.

The approaches managers can take to the fact that things can go wrong in their programs or projects are conceptually similar to what clinicians do regarding the safety of their patients. In both instances, clinicians and managers focus on *preventing* things from going wrong. However, when something does go wrong, the focus shifts to *containing and minimizing* the damage. Finally, the focus becomes one of *addressing* the consequences of negative occurrences.

In seeking to prevent mishaps, contain and minimize the resulting damage from them, and address the consequences of them, managers engage in different activities, although ideally the activities are integrated. Throughout, communicating plays a vital role. Each set of activities managers use to manage and communicate about things going wrong is considered next.

Preventing Things from Going Wrong

In attempting to prevent the occurrence of negative events managers are increasingly turning to integrated sets of activities aimed at making certain that the right things are done, that they are done correctly, and that they are done correctly the first time (Deming 1986; Juran 1989; Griffith and White 2002). As is discussed more fully in Chapter Seven, these sets of activities go by various names. A popular one is *continuous quality improvement* or CQI. James (1989) suggests that the essence of CQI is to answer three questions: Are we doing the right things? Are we doing things right? How can we be certain that we do things right the first time, every time? In Chapter Seven, we label these integrated sets of activities *total quality* (TQ) and discuss the approach extensively. Each of these sets of activities relies heavily upon communications.

By whatever name they are called, these substantial and organized efforts focus on continuous improvement in performance (including preventing negative occurrences), and provide a framework within which undesirable events, at least those under the control of managers, can be avoided or minimized. The framework works best in combination with activities designed to reduce risk and reap the benefits of organizational learning (Senge 1990). Although there is no way to avoid all unwanted occurrences, such as errors in patient care, concerted efforts can help reduce the frequency and severity in health programs and projects.

Containing and Minimizing the Damage

No matter how hard managers work to prevent it, and no matter what means they employ to this end, things will go wrong in health programs and projects. The focus then becomes one of containing and minimizing the damage. In seeking to do this, managers engage in activities that are guided by concepts and models of assessing and controlling performance. (The reader may wish to review the section on this topic in Chapter Two.)

In controlling, managers seek to assure that the processes used in their domains, as well as the outputs, outcomes, and impact achieved in their domains, are continuously monitored, that the results are assessed, and, when necessary, that interventions are undertaken to contain the damage caused by something going wrong. In addition, the CQI or TQ programs and the risk-management programs instituted to prevent problems also include elements intended to help contain the damage when such events occur.

In exerting control, managers seek to regulate activities and events in accordance with pre-established plans and standards. When control is exercised effectively, deviations from established standards are noticed quickly and corrective actions are taken to curb the damage that might otherwise be done. Both the detection of deviations and the corrective responses rely upon managers and other participants communicating effectively.

However, the reality is that when prevention fails, regardless of how effectively the resulting damage has been contained, some damage will have been done. As noted previously, damage done in health programs and projects often has significant direct and indirect consequences for both internal and external stakeholders. When things go wrong, the manager's focus eventually shifts to addressing the consequences.

Addressing the Consequences

Before anything constructive can be done to address the consequences of something going wrong in a program or project, those who suffer the consequences must be identified. Sometimes this is easily done. Patients/customers who are harmed, their families, participants who are injured on the job or who are laid off from their work, and their families endure obvious consequences. Less obviously perhaps, potential patients/customers and other participants who learn of such events and feel less positively about a program or project are also experiencing consequences. Stores and restaurants feel the ripple effects of a program or project's termination when they lose customers.

Indeed, when something goes wrong in a health program or project, there may be consequences for many individuals, groups, and organizations. Collectively, the people and organizations who might be harmed when things go wrong are the same as those who stand to benefit when things go right–the program or project's internal and external stakeholders. The best way for managers to fully understand and appreciate the consequences of events for stakeholders is through communicating with them, or at least with representative samples of them.

Once those directly or indirectly affected have been identified, the ethically sound goal of fully addressing the consequences of a negative event requires restoring positions and conditions as closely as possible to positions and conditions extant before the event. Achieving this goal across the board may not be possible (some wrongs can never be righted), but it is the appropriate goal and should guide decisions and actions, including how the manager communicates with the stakeholders.

Each instance of something going wrong requires its own unique set of decisions and actions to appropriately manage the event's consequences. There are few hard-and-fast rules to guide managers in developing these sets of decisions and actions, although their potential decisions and actions range along a rather clear-cut continuum of appropriateness, as illustrated in Figure 6.9.

At one end of the continuum, the most inappropriate responses are characterized by attempts to conceal the fact that something has gone wrong–by doing and communicating as little as possible about what has happened or, in the extreme, by telling lies and misleading others about what has happened. Somewhat less extreme is to respond by acknowledging that something has gone wrong, but to deny wrongdoing, avoid or minimize responsibility, and take no action to address the consequences. Guided by a preference for this type of response, a program or project's manager most likely will take an obstructionist approach regarding the event and communicate about it only minimally.

FIGURE 6.9. MANAGEMENT APPROACHES WHEN SOMETHING GOES WRONG.

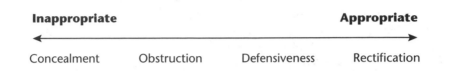

Inappropriate			Appropriate
Concealment	Obstruction	Defensiveness	Rectification

A third type of response to something going wrong is labeled defensiveness. The manager (or another spokesperson) follows the letter of the law when taking action or communicating about what has gone wrong. This is a common response to serious negative events and reflects the intention to minimize legal liability. Decisions and actions based on this approach may be entirely legal, but they also can be far from the ethical high ground.

A defensive approach to dealing with the consequences of an untoward event partly reflects how expensive taking responsibility can be. Serious problems involving human health and life can be very expensive. However, a defensive approach may be taken even when the issues are layoffs, program or project service reductions or terminations, or other operational problems that affect internal or external stakeholders. Managers can find themselves conflicted between fully addressing the consequences of untoward events and preserving the program or project's financial assets, good name, and reputation. But the defensive position, so often occupied when something goes wrong, falls short of the most appropriate response.

At the most appropriate end of the continuum in Figure 6.9 is a type of response called *rectification*. Rectification is characterized by accepting responsibility for what has gone wrong and undertaking aggressive actions to address the consequences for and rectify the harms to all those who have been affected, including communicating extensively with them.

Managers who pursue a rectification response take a positive and proactive stance toward addressing the negative consequences. Their decisions and resultant actions reflect this stance. Communications are characterized by openness and candor about what went wrong, its causes, and the actions being taken to deal with the consequences.

The pattern of a program or project's responses to things going wrong builds upon itself. Responses characterized by concealment, obstruction, and to a large extent, defensiveness, once detected by stakeholders, increase distrust and invite intensified scrutiny of the immediate situation and of similar future situations. In contrast, programs and projects with established histories of undertaking rectification responses when things go wrong build trust among their stakeholders.

With such histories, little or no effort is wasted by stakeholders wondering whether they are being provided all relevant information about a negative event or about the program or project manager's determination to fully address its consequences. The payoff for the program or project that behaves in this way includes an easier and faster return to a suitable equilibrium with its stakeholders after the untoward event.

Obviously, the best way to manage negative events in health programs and projects is to prevent their occurrence. Carefully orchestrated CQI or TQ efforts can be very beneficial in preventing or minimizing the occurrence of problems. When prevention fails, however, managers must turn their attention to containing the damage that flows from unwanted events and to addressing their consequences. In this, managers are best served by aggressive, positive, and proactive efforts to identify the harmed stakeholders and to return them as closely as possible to the positions and conditions they experienced before the event, and to communicate with them openly and extensively in doing so.

Summary

Communicating involves senders, who can be individuals, groups, or organizations, conveying ideas, intentions, and information to receivers, who can also be individuals, groups, or organizations. Communication is effective when receivers understand ideas, intentions, or information as senders intend.

Communication is not restricted to words; it includes all methods (verbal and nonverbal) through which meaning is conveyed. The technical process of communication is modeled in Figure 6.3. Particular attention is given to describing the contextual and interpersonal barriers to effective communication and to the means available to managers for overcoming the barriers.

Managers must be concerned with two basic types of communications: those internal to the program or project, and those with external stakeholders. Communication within programs and projects depends on formal channels and networks to transmit information and understanding in all directions and on widespread acknowledgement of the existence and effective use of these channels. The channels carry information downward, upward, horizontally, and diagonally and have characteristics that make them useful for the purposes illustrated in Figure 6.4. Coexisting with formal communication flows are informal flows that consist of channels and networks (the grapevine) that arise from the interpersonal relationships among the participants in programs and projects.

Increasingly, managers are concerned with communications between their programs or projects and external stakeholders. Effective formal and informal communication flows to and from external stakeholders are important to successfully managing programs and projects. Examples of effective communication flows include marketing a program's services; monitoring regulatory changes in government agencies that might affect a project; or lobbying for more favorable reimbursement rates for services provided by a program.

Chapter Review Questions

1. Define communicating and draw a model of the basic communicating process.
2. Describe both contextual and interpersonal barriers to communicating effectively in programs and projects, and identify ways these barriers can be managed.
3. Describe the flows of communication within health programs and projects and give an example of each type of flow.
4. Describe three common communication networks and give an example of each type.
5. Discuss the role of informal communication in programs and projects.
6. Identify two especially important external stakeholders for programs and projects and discuss effective ways to communicate with them.
7. Discuss the role of communication with both internal and external stakeholders when something goes wrong in a health program or project.

CHAPTER SEVEN

MANAGING QUALITY—TOTALLY

Managers in health programs and projects typically give high priority to the quality of services provided. Quality is also important to other participants in programs and projects. For example, it has been clearly established that people who work in settings that strive to continuously improve quality find higher levels of satisfaction from their work (Berlowitz and others 2003). Furthermore, quality is also important to recipients of a program or project's services and often influences their future service-seeking decisions.

Managing quality well is among the most challenging management responsibilities. A major study conducted within the British National Health Services suggests some of the reasons for the challenge of managing quality well, including "the inertia built into established ways of working, and the effort needed to implement new work processes" (Ham, Kipping, and McLeod 2003, p. 434).

The Institute of Medicine has given a great deal of attention to the issue of quality and safety in health care, as reflected in their list of ten things patients/customers should be able to expect from providers of health services, no matter what the setting. Clearly an ideal to be pursued, these expectations (listed in Figure 7.1) suggest the difficulty of fully meeting the challenges of satisfying contemporary patients/customers regarding the quality and safety of their health services.

The challenge of managing quality is substantial, and there is much room for improvement in efforts to meet the challenge. Participants in the National Roundtable on Health Care Quality convened by the Institute of Medicine concluded that, "At its best, health care in the United States is superb. Unfortunately,

FIGURE 7.1. WHAT PATIENTS/CUSTOMERS SHOULD EXPECT OF HEALTH CARE SERVICES.

1. **Beyond patient visits:** You will have the care you need when you need it . . . whenever you need it. You will find help in many forms, not just in face-to-face visits. You will find help on the Internet, on the telephone, from many sources, by many routes, in the form you want it.

2. **Individualization:** You will be known and respected as an individual. Your choices and preferences will be sought and honored. The usual system of care will meet most of your needs. When your needs are special, the care will adapt to meet you on your own terms.

3. **Control:** The care system will take control only if and when you freely give permission.

4. **Information:** You can know what you wish to know, when you wish to know it. Your medical record is yours to keep, to read, and to understand. The rule is: "Nothing about you without you."

5. **Science:** You will have care based on the best available scientific knowledge. The system promises you excellence as its standard. Your care will not vary illogically from doctor to doctor or from place to place. The system will promise you all the care that can help you, and will help you avoid care that cannot help you.

6. **Safety:** Errors in care will not harm you. You will be safe in the care system.

7. **Transparency:** Your care will be confidential, but the care system will not keep secrets from you. You can know whatever you wish to know about the care that affects you and your loved ones.

8. **Anticipation:** Your care will anticipate your needs and will help you find the help you need. You will experience proactive help, not just reactions, to help you restore and maintain your health.

9. **Value:** Your care will not waste your time or money. You will benefit from constant innovations, which will increase the value of care to you.

10. **Cooperation:** Those who provide care will cooperate and coordinate their work fully with each other and with you. The walls between professions and institutions will crumble, so that your experiences will become seamless. You will never feel lost.

Source: Reprinted with permission from *Crossing the Quality Chasm: A New Health System for the 21st Century*, p. 63. © 2001 by the National Academy of Sciences. Courtesy of the National Academy Press, Washington, D.C.

it is often not at its best. Problems in health care quality are serious and extensive; they occur in all delivery systems and financing mechanisms. Americans bear a great burden of harm because of these problems, a burden that is measured in lost lives, reduced functioning, and wasted resources. Collectively, these problems call for urgent action" (Institute of Medicine 1998, p. 11).

After defining quality as it applies to health services and describing its measurement, a framework called a *total quality (TQ) approach* to the systematic management of quality in health programs and projects is presented. The framework includes three interconnected principles: a patient/customer focus, the implementation of continuous improvement activities, and teamwork. These principles can guide efforts to manage quality in all programs and projects. After reading the chapter, the reader should be able to do the following:

- Define quality of health services and describe the two components of quality
- Understand structural, process, and outcome measures of quality
- Understand the TQ approach to managing quality
- Understand the application of the three principles that underpin the TQ approach: patient/customer focus, continuous improvement, and teamwork

Quality Defined

Quality of health services has been defined by the Institute of Medicine as "the degree to which health services for individuals and populations increase the likelihood of desired health outcomes and are consistent with current professional knowledge" (Institute of Medicine 1990, p. 21). There are, of course, many other definitions of quality as it applies to health care and to health services. Most definitions have been influenced by the paradigm established by Avedis Donabedian (1980) that describes the dual nature of quality in terms of its technical and interpersonal components. More recently, in an analysis that reviewed many definitions of quality, researchers concluded that most definitions reflect two components of quality: technical quality and treating people in a humane and culturally appropriate manner (Brook, McGlynn, and Shekelle 2000). These authors use high technical quality to mean that "the patient receives only the procedures, tests, or services, for which the desired health outcomes exceed the health risks by a sufficiently wide margin and . . . each of these procedures or services is performed in a technically excellent manner." The authors define the second component of quality of care to be "that all patients wish to be treated in a humane and culturally appropriate manner and be invited to participate fully in deciding about their therapy" (Brook, McGlynn, and Shekelle 2000, p. 282).

An individual's value system and the conditions and circumstances confronting an individual in a particular situation influence which component is more important to the person. People with immediate and acute concerns, such as whether or not they are HIV positive, may be primarily interested in the technical expertise of those doing the testing. Whereas people with chronic conditions, such as well-controlled diabetes, may be more concerned about being treated humanely and in a culturally sensitive manner over a long period of time.

James (1989) has characterized the two components as (1) *content quality* and (2) *delivery and service quality*. By content quality, he means the clinical expertise and technical aspects of providing health services. By delivery and service quality, he means the interpersonal aspects of service provision such as empathy, communication, and how well the patients/customers' requirements and expectations are being met for such things as convenience and timeliness. For managers of health programs and projects, both components of quality are relevant and must be addressed.

Measuring Quality

From a management perspective, the measurement of quality, including both its technical and interpersonal components, is requisite to managing and improving the level of quality of the services provided in a program or project. Sometimes called quality assessment, the measurement of quality has its origins in the work of Donabedian (1980), who pointed out that the measurement of quality includes *structural measures* (innate characteristics of those who provide services and of the settings in which they are provided); *process measures* (what service providers do to patients/customers); and *outcome measures* (what happens to the health of patients/customers as a result of services).

Structural measures of quality in a health program or project are measures of available inputs and resources that can be associated with quality. These measures include indicators such as the number and credentials of staff, presence of specialized state-of-the-art equipment, use of active peer review, and accreditation or approval by outside agencies. Process measures include indicators of compliance to protocols, such as the percentage of elderly patients/customers served who appropriately receive an influenza vaccine or whether children served receive the immunizations they need when they need them. Outcome measures include indicators that reflect changes in patients' or customers' health status and level of satisfaction. These are "bottom line" measures of how well health services delivery works. Outcomes often include such clinical indicators as mortality and functional health status, and they also include levels of patient/customer satisfaction.

The National Quality Measures Clearinghouse (NQMC), which is sponsored by the Agency for Healthcare Quality and Research (AHRQ), maintains a Web site (http://www.qualitymeasures.ahrq.gov) containing extensive information on specific evidence-based quality measures and measure sets. Another Web site maintained by AHRQ is for the National Guideline Clearinghouse (NGC) (http://www.guidelines.gov). This Web site contains a comprehensive database of evidence-based clinical practice guidelines produced by AHRQ in partnership with the American Medical Association (AMA) and the American Association of Health Plans (AAHP).

Managing Quality

Assuring quality and safety in health programs and projects cannot be separated from other management work. For example, the presence of five specific management practices is associated with a greater likelihood that a program or project will achieve higher levels of quality and safety. These practices are: (1) achieving a balance between requirements for productivity and for quality and safety, (2) establishing and maintaining trust among participants, (3) managing the process of change effectively, (4) permitting high levels of participation by the program or project's participants in decision making about the logic model and organization design, and (5) operating the program or project as a learning organization (Page 2004, p. 107).

Above all else, managing quality in a program or project requires a *systematic* approach. Over the years, several different systematic approaches to quality in delivery of health services have been taken. These are best viewed as steps in an evolutionary process leading to the contemporary approaches.

One early approach to managing quality was *quality assurance* (QA), which has been described as a formal and systematic exercise of identifying problems in health care delivery, and of designing and implementing means to resolve these problems (Brook and Lohr 1985). In essence, QA is a process of eliminating defects (Kelly 2003), and as such is a negative process (Longest, Rakich, and Darr 2000).

Supplanting the QA approach in the 1990s, *quality improvement* (QI) arose as a more positive and broader approach to managing quality. This approach builds upon the work of such industrial quality experts as Crosby (1989), Deming (1982), and Juran (1989). QI has also been called *continuous quality improvement,* or CQI (McLaughlin and Kaluzny 1994). James (1989) suggests the essence of the CQI approach to quality is to answer three questions: Are we doing the right things? Are we doing things right? How can we be certain that we do things right the first time, every time?

Contemporary approaches to quality tend to be conceptually broad and to reflect a management philosophy. These approaches have been called *quality management* (James 1989; Kelly 2003); *total quality management,* or TQM, (McLaughlin and Kaluzny 1990); or simply *total quality,* or TQ (Dean and Bowen 1994). Although the variety of terms can be confusing, these newer systematic approaches to quality are characterized by the application of similar principles, practices, and techniques.

A Total Quality (TQ) Approach to Managing Quality

Three *principles* guide managers in the pursuit of a TQ approach to managing quality in health programs and projects: patient/customer focus, continuous improvement, and teamwork (Dean and Bowen 1994). Figure 7.2 illustrates the interconnected nature of the principles that underpin a TQ approach.

The principle of *patient/customer focus* requires managers in pursuit of quality to identify what a program or project's patients/customers need and want, and then to design and deliver services that satisfy those needs and wants. The principle of *continuous improvement* requires managers to make a commitment to search for better ways to provide services through continuously examining and refining the processes through which services are provided. Finally, the principle of *teamwork,* because TQ is a collective responsibility of all those involved in a program or project, requires a collaborative effort in pursuit of TQ. Teams are by definition collections of individuals who share interdependent tasks and responsibility for outcomes or results (Cohen and Bailey 1997; LaFasto and Larson 2001).

The patient/customer focus, continuous improvement, and teamwork triad of a TQ approach can be used in the smallest program or project, or in the largest

FIGURE 7.2. THE GUIDING PRINCIPLES OF THE TOTAL QUALITY (TQ) APPROACH.

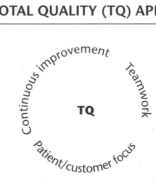

corporation. For example, Intel Corporation treats quality as one of its core values and says, "The quest for total quality delivers a wealth of advantages to Intel and customers alike. High-quality timely products and services not only help our customers succeed, but also reduce our cost of doing business and steadily increase our market share" (Intel Corporation 2003, p. 1-1). GE, one of the world's largest and most successful corporations, says that customer, process, and employee are the key elements of quality and that "Everything we do to remain a world-class quality company focuses on these three essential elements" (http://www.ge.com/sixsigma/keyelements.html). Each of the three principles underlying a TQ approach to managing quality—patient/customer focus, continuous improvement, and teamwork—is described in more detail in the following sections.

Focusing on Patients/Customers

The purpose of focusing on patients/customers is to make certain services that satisfy their wants and needs are designed and delivered. Satisfaction of patients/ customers is a vital element in the long-term success of any program or project. The prominent place of this focus in the selection criteria for the Malcolm Baldrige National Quality Award Program attests to the centrality of focusing on patients/ customers in achieving overall performance excellence in health programs and projects (National Institute of Standards and Technology 2003).

The Baldrige Award was created when the United States enacted the Malcolm Baldrige National Quality Improvement Act of 1987 (Public Law 100-107) for the purpose, as stated in the act, "of encouraging American business and other organizations to practice effective quality control in the provision of their goods and services." The Award is named for Malcolm Baldrige, who served as Secretary of Commerce from 1981 until his death in 1987. His managerial excellence contributed to long-term improvement in efficiency and effectiveness of government. The President of the United States presents the Baldrige Award annually to competitively selected business, education, and health care organizations in recognition of significant achievements in quality and performance excellence.

The award criteria, which can be read at http://www.quality.nist.gov/ HealthCare_Criteria.htm, are intended to encourage managers to take an integrated approach to performance management that results in "delivery of ever-improving value to patients and other customers, contributing to improved health care quality" (National Institute of Standards and Technology 2003, p. 1). Figure 7.3 summarizes the questions asked of candidates for the Baldrige Award to document their approach to patient/customer relationships and satisfaction. Answering these questions can be useful to any manager interested in establishing a patient/customer focus in a program or project.

FIGURE 7.3. DOCUMENTING A PATIENT/CUSTOMER FOCUS IN THE BALDRIGE NATIONAL QUALITY AWARD.

Describe HOW your organization builds relationships to acquire, satisfy, and retain PATIENTS and other CUSTOMERS; to increase loyalty; and to develop new HEALTH CARE SERVICE opportunities. Describe also HOW your organization determines PATIENT and other CUSTOMER satisfaction.

Within your response, include answers to the following questions:

A. PATIENT/CUSTOMER Relationship Building

1. How do you build relationships to acquire PATIENTS and other CUSTOMERS, to meet and exceed their expectations, to increase loyalty and secure their future interactions with your organization, and to gain positive referrals?

2. What are your KEY access mechanisms for PATIENTS and other CUSTOMERS to seek information, obtain services, and make complaints? How do you determine KEY contact requirements for each mode of PATIENT and other CUSTOMER access? How do you ensure that these contact requirements are deployed to all people and PROCESSES involved in the CUSTOMER response chain?

3. What is your complaint management PROCESS? How do you ensure that complaints are resolved effectively and promptly? How are complaints aggregated and analyzed for use in improvement throughout your organization and by your partners?

4. How do you keep your APPROACHES to building relationships and providing PATIENT/CUSTOMER access current with HEALTH CARE SERVICE needs and directions?

B. PATIENT/CUSTOMER Satisfaction Determination

1. How do you determine PATIENT and other CUSTOMER satisfaction and dissatisfaction? How do these determination methods differ among PATIENT/CUSTOMER groups? How do you ensure that your measurements capture actionable information for use in exceeding your PATIENTS' and other CUSTOMERS' expectations, securing their future interactions with your organization, and gaining positive referrals? How do you use PATIENT and other CUSTOMER satisfaction and dissatisfaction information for improvement?

2. How do you follow up with PATIENTS and other CUSTOMERS on HEALTH CARE SERVICES and transaction quality to receive prompt and actionable feedback?

3. How do you obtain and use information on PATIENTS' and other CUSTOMERS' satisfaction relative to satisfaction with your competitors, other organizations providing similar HEALTH CARE SERVICES, and/or BENCHMARKS?

4. How do you keep your APPROACHES to determining satisfaction current with HEALTH CARE SERVICE needs and directions?

Source: National Institute of Standards and Technology, *Healthcare Criteria for Performance Excellence,* Washington, D.C.: National Institute of Standards and Technology, 2003, p. 23. Used with permission of the National Institute of Standards and Technology.

An effective patient/customer focus requires first that patients/customers be carefully identified. As is discussed fully in Chapter Eight, in the section on commercial marketing, health programs and projects can have many different customers. Patients, along with their families and significant others, are obvious customers. So, too, are potential patients and their families. The positions in a program or project's organization design must be staffed with appropriate participants. Thus, employees and potential employees are customers. As noted earlier, employees typically prefer to work in settings that strive to continuously improve quality (Berlowitz and others 2003). Similarly, volunteers are more likely to be attracted to programs and projects they perceive to be of high quality. Programs and projects that rely on donors for partial financial support must treat them as customers in TQ activities. Some programs and projects may need to satisfy public and private payers like Medicaid programs or insurance plans as to their quality. Successful programs or projects often depend on physicians or other health care providers to refer patients, which makes the providers important customers. When programs and projects are embedded in larger organizations, it is important to assure the host organization of the quality of the program or project. Indeed, there are many customers to be considered in a TQ approach.

Although a TQ approach focuses on all customers, patients and other customers who receive services are typically the primary focus for health programs and projects. After all, the provision of services to patients/customers is the principle reason such programs or projects exist. Studies using focus groups of patients and other research methods document that patients want their health services to be of high technical quality and to contain an appropriate interpersonal component (Gerteis, Edgman-Levitan, Daley, and Delbanco 2002). Inclusion of an appropriate interpersonal component requires that attention be given to the following:

- Patients' and customers' values and preferences
- Patients' and customers' physical comfort, including pain control
- Patients' and customers' emotional and psychological comfort, including alleviation of fear and anxiety
- Patients' and customers' need for information from and open communication with those who provide services

Continuous Improvement

The second principle of a TQ approach to managing quality is continuous improvement (CI). Underpinning this principle is the concept that it is through continuously improving the processes inherent in programs and projects' logic models that the needs and wants of patients/customers can be more completely met. Certainly, in the complex processes through which health services are provided there are many opportunities for improvement. These opportunities are inherent in goals for perfection in health care. For example, Chassin (1998) states such goals as follows:

- Always providing effective health services to those who could benefit from them
- Always avoiding the provision of ineffective health services
- Eliminating all preventable complications in the health services that are provided

Realistically, absolute perfection is not attainable in the provision of health services in any setting. However, contemporary quality improvement efforts are increasingly establishing goals that approach perfection. One of the most popular ways of expressing such goals in corporations (such as Motorola, GE, IBM, American Express, and many others) has been their adoption of a *Six Sigma* approach to CI. Health care organizations, including programs and projects, are beginning to move in this direction as well (Barry, Murcko, and Brubaker 2002).

Sigma is a statistical term meaning standard deviation, and in application to CI can be used to measure how far a given process deviates from perfection. Technically, the statistical term, six sigma, from which the Six Sigma approach draws its name, simply means that in a process governed by a normal distribution, values more than six standard deviations away from the average will occur only 3.4 times in a million opportunities. This is a very small number and in a practical application to QI means that errors in a process would occur only 3.4 times in a million opportunities. While not perfection, this is very close to it.

The central idea behind Six Sigma is that if the number of defects or errors existing in a process can be measured, then steps can be taken to move the process as close to zero defects as possible. Six Sigma is data-driven and relies on extensive use of statistical analysis. As Revere and Black (2003) note, Six Sigma complements, embellishes, and expands TQ, especially in that the goals developed in the Six Sigma approach are very aggressive. A great deal of information about Six Sigma is available at http://www.isixsigma.com for the interested reader. Adopters of the Six Sigma approach to CI typically follow eight steps in their efforts to improve performance:

Step 1.   Identify critical processes where improved performance is important.
Step 2.   Quantify present performance by measurement and statistical analysis to serve as a baseline.
Step 3.   Consider possible changes to improve the process.
Step 4.   Implement changes on a trial basis.

Step 5.   Monitor and assess the implementation experience.

Step 6.   Extend and make permanent successful changes.

Step 7.   Monitor the new process on an ongoing basis to assure stability.

Step 8.   Identify the next process for improvement and repeat the cycle.

Another popular contemporary approach to CI is the *Toyota Production System,* or TPS. Over many years, the Toyota Motor Manufacturing Corporation developed a set of principles that facilitate a self-reflective process involving designing, testing, and improving work so all participants contribute at or near their full potential. Spear and Bowen observe that "Toyota uses a rigorous problem-solving process that requires a detailed assessment of the current state of affairs and a plan for improvement that is, in effect, an experimental test of the proposed changes" (1999, p. 98). These authors also describe the principles that underlie TPS, noting that this approach to CI is built upon ideas about how people work, how they connect with other people in performing work, and how production processes are best set up. Above all else, in their view, the success of TPS is based upon teaching all participants how to use the scientific method in pursuing improvement.

Although Six Sigma and TPS incorporate unique features, they are based upon the fundamental conceptual approach underlying all comprehensive CI efforts, an approach that is described in the next section.

The FOCUS-PDCA Model.   The most widely used CI model is *FOCUS-PDCA.* Figure 7.4 shows the complete FOCUS-PDCA model. The FOCUS part of the acronym derives from the following:

Find a process to improve.

Organize an improvement team and necessary resources.

Clarify current knowledge about the process.

Understand the process and sources of variation in it.

Select an improvement or intervention.

The PDCA part of the acronym is based on a model developed by Walter A. Shewhart at Bell Laboratories in the 1930s. Shewhart observed that constant evaluation of processes was essential to CI, along with the willingness of managers to adopt or disregard changes in the processes based on evidence of their utility. In what has come to be called the *Shewhart Cycle,* he developed the plan-do-check-act (PDCA) cycle to guide managers in their efforts to make process improvements by first planning an action intended to improve a process based

FIGURE 7.4. FOCUS-PDCA MODEL.

Step 1: **F**ind a process to improve.

Step 2: **O**rganize an improvement team and necessary resources.

Step 3: **C**larify current knowledge about the process.

Step 4: **U**nderstand the process and sources of variation in it.

Step 5: **S**elect an improvement or intervention.

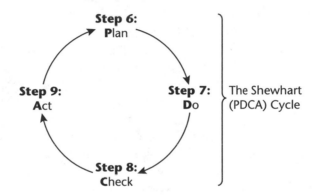

on careful study of the process, then implementing the action on a small scale, then checking to see how results conform to the plan, and then acting on what has been learned as follows:

Plan how to implement the intervention.

Do it by initiating the intervention, often on a small scale at first.

Check the results of the early implementation, revising as necessary, until it proves itself as an improvement.

Act on what was learned in the check step. If the change was successful, incorporate it on a larger scale and make it permanent. If the change wasn't successful, go through the cycle again with a different plan.

An example of the application of the FOCUS-PDCA model is the work of a CI team established in a family practice program attempting to improve the care of people with type 2 diabetes using the model as a guide (Schwarz, Landis, and Rowe 1999). This CI team proceeded through the steps in Figure 7.4 as follows:

Step 1. Find a process to improve. The program's CI efforts began, as many do, with consideration of how their processes compare to so-called best practices. The program wanted to be certain that the care of their patients measured up to the best practice standards in caring for patients with type 2 diabetes. In effect, the program used one of the most basic of CI tools, *benchmarking,* as a means of identifying a process to improve. Unless current performance of a process measures up to the benchmark, it is a candidate for improvement.

Benchmarking is a process whereby those pursuing CI establish operating targets based on leading performance standards for particular processes. Benchmarks are more than mere metrics against which to judge performance. In application, benchmarking is a philosophy that guides CI activities toward the goal of achieving the best possible performance in processes. This is accomplished through emulating the performance levels achieved by those who perform processes in an exemplary or benchmark manner. Steps in applying benchmarking include identifying who or what to benchmark, collecting information on best practice standards, and using the information to guide CI efforts.

Step 2. Organize an improvement team and necessary resources. The CI team was formed based on each member's knowledge of the process to be improved. The members were a physician, a nurse, and a laboratory technician. A representative from the business office served as a consultant to the team. The physician member was the team leader, and another member who had been trained as a facilitator served as facilitator. (More information on teams and teamwork is provided in a subsequent section in this chapter.)

Step 3. Clarify current knowledge about the process. The CI team conducted a literature review to gather information about appropriate clinical guidelines for the care of patients with diabetes, then collected and reviewed data about the program's patients. In the literature review, they focused on the process through which patients with type 2 diabetes are seen in well-run programs, and became especially interested in whether their patients were receiving appropriate HbA_{1c} tests. (The HbA_{1c} test is an excellent way to monitor blood sugar levels in patients over three-month periods.)

In order to establish a baseline of information in their own program, the team identified all patients who had the type 2 diabetes diagnosis during the past year. The team audited a random sample of these patients' charts to determine the program's rate of ordering HbA_{1c} tests, as well as the average HbA_{1c} value. After reviewing the results, the team decided they could improve diabetes management by increasing the number of patients who received at least two HbA_{1c} tests per year

Step 4. Understand the process and sources of variation in it. The processes through which health services are provided are composed of operations, steps, or activities through which people, material, or information flows. One of the most useful ways to understand a process is to carefully document or chart it to identify places where improvements can be made. W*orkflow charting* involves establishing the boundaries of a process, identifying the steps in the process and their sequence, and showing the flow of people, material, or information.

Figure 7.5 is a workflow chart developed by the CI team to help them understand the care process for patients with diabetes. Flowcharts use symbols to illustrate what happens in each step of a process. For example, a parallelogram represents the starting point, a rectangle represents a task or activity performed during the process, a diamond represents a yes-no decision point, and an oval represents the end point of the process.

Step 5. Select an improvement or intervention. Based on the previous steps, the CI team decided that a potentially useful intervention was to attach a reminder form to the first page of the medical record at every encounter with patients who had been diagnosed with type 2 diabetes. This form provided guidelines on the frequency of tests and procedures to improve care of these patients. The form and its use was the team's selected intervention.

Step 6. Plan how to implement the intervention. The planning step is vital to a successful implementation of any intervention or improvement. To implement the use of diabetes care reminders, the CI team found that the office, nursing, and laboratory staff, as well as physicians, needed instructions about how to use the new reminders. They also had to decide who would print out the reminders, who would ensure they were attached to the first page of the medical records, and who would enter the laboratory values on them. All of this required careful planning.

Step 7. Do it by initiating the intervention, even if on a small scale at first. The CI team initiated the intervention by having the reminder forms attached to all medical records for all encounters with patients with the diabetes diagnosis, and by encouraging the use of the reminder forms.

Step 8. Check the results of the early implementation. It is important that interventions be monitored to determine if they are having the desired effect. This step may trigger necessary revisions before an improvement is considered completely developed. In checking on whether their intervention was improving diabetes care, the CI team was able to track changes in the frequency of ordering HbA_{1c} tests.

FIGURE 7.5. PRE-INTERVENTION FLOWCHART
OF PATIENT CARE PROCESS.

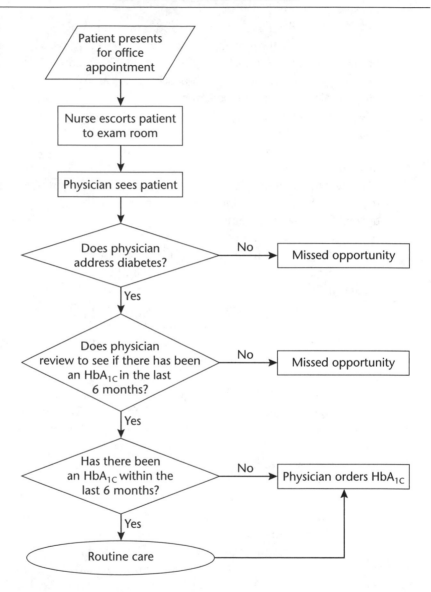

Step 9. Act on what was learned in the check step. If an intervention or change is successful, the CI team can incorporate it on a larger scale and make it permanent. If not, they can go through the cycle again with a different plan. The diabetes care CI team was very pleased with the intervention and the improvement in care for patients. They gave each physician in the program individualized and program-wide data on HbA_{1c} performance, and celebrated their success with a catered lunch.

Looking to the future, the team established goals that 80 percent of the program's patients with type 2 diabetes would have all tests and procedures completed (and documented on the reminder form) and that 80 percent would have their most recent HbA_{1c} values at less than 7.5 percent. To meet these goals, the diabetes team planned to explore additional interventions including automatic HbA_{1c} reminders for patients and educational support-group sessions for patients.

Step 9 reflects that CI is an ongoing process. What teams learn in one round of CI can inform and broaden the results of that round and can stimulate participants to look for other aspects of processes to improve.

Whether an approach to CI is called Six Sigma, Toyota Production System, FOCUS-PDCA, or something else, effective *systematic* approaches to process improvement all share the common characteristic that they begin with diagnosing something about a process that needs to be changed and extend through to the implementation and evaluation of changes that are made in processes. The steps are similar to the steps routinely taken in managing changes. Longest (1998b), for example, describes these steps as identification, planning and preparation, implementation, and evaluation. The steps in a CI approach are also similar to the general approach to making good management decisions discussed in Chapter Five (see Figure 5.2).

Tools for CI. In addition to *benchmarking* and *workflow charting* noted previously, several additional tools are useful in conducting CI activities, especially in determining what should be changed about a process in order to improve it. One of the simplest and most useful tools is a *cause-and-effect diagram* or, as it is popularly known because of its shape, a *fishbone diagram*. The fishbone pattern is readily visible in Figure 7.6, a generalized cause-and-effect diagram. The reader may wish to review Figure 5.3, which is a specific example of the application of a cause-and-effect diagram.

Use of this diagram in determining the possible causes of a problem in a process and in deciding what can be done to improve the process is based on organizing the examination or study of the process. Is the problem caused by

FIGURE 7.6. A GENERALIZED FISHBONE
OR CAUSE-AND-EFFECT DIAGRAM.

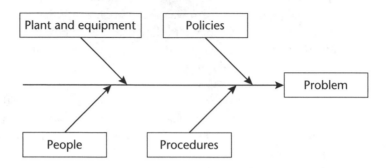

something people are doing or not doing? Is it a matter of inadequate equipment or poor layout of physical space? Perhaps the problem is caused in part by a confusing policy or an incomplete procedural protocol. A carefully constructed fishbone diagram of the potential causes of a problem often yields multiple causes or process variables that can be changed to improve the process.

Because problems may have numerous underlying causes, another useful tool in CI is a *Pareto diagram* or chart, which is a bar graph that can show the relative importance of elements in a process that contribute to a problem. For example, the Pareto diagram depicted in Figure 5.4, which the reader may wish to review, shows the relative importance of process variables in causing cases of nosocomial pneumonia. In that instance, a Pareto analysis determined that relatively few variables caused most of the problem. These few variables became the focus of efforts to improve the process.

A *run chart,* which is a graphic representation of data over time, can be very useful in monitoring the progress of a CI intervention and in confirming that the intervention actually led to improvement. Figure 7.7 is a run chart of average patient waiting times before and after an intervention designed to shorten waiting times.

This run chart shows that for several months prior to the intervention, the average waiting times increased for the patients in a program. Following the intervention the average waiting times declined for subsequent months, indicating that the intervention had the desired effect and improved this process.

Additional information about CI and tools to support it can be found at the Web site of the Institute for Healthcare Improvement (http://www.ihi.org). IHI is a not-for-profit organization devoted to improving the delivery of health services. Another useful resource is the Institute for Clinical Systems Improvement (http://www.icsi.org). ICSI is a collaboration of health care organizations also devoted to improving the delivery of health services by helping its members identify and accelerate implementation of best clinical practices for their patients/customers.

Teamwork

The third principle of a TQ approach to managing quality is teamwork. Most significant improvements in processes that lead to better quality are accomplished by teams rather than by individuals. Teams and teamwork are essential to successful TQ approaches. For example, it has been demonstrated that quality improvement activities increase in nursing home settings with cultures that emphasize teamwork (Berlowitz and others 2003). As noted previously, the emphasis on teamwork reflects that participants in a program or project share *collective* responsibility for CI when a TQ approach is being taken.

Collaborative effort in TQ approaches typically occurs in the context of *improvement teams*. Such teams can be formed to address specific problems or issues, or they can be formed for the more general purpose of improving performance in particular areas. In some situations, all participants in a program or project are thought of as a team. In other situations, smaller groups of participants form teams. In both cases, teams are collections of participants who share interdependent tasks, as well as responsibility for outcomes or results.

FIGURE 7.7. RUN CHART OF INTERVENTION TO SHORTEN WAITING TIMES.

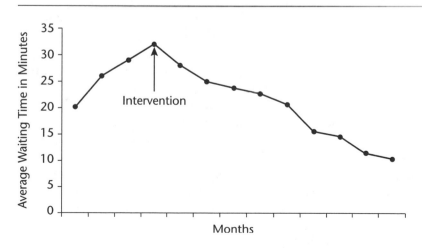

Managers *design* effective teams; effective teams do not just form spontaneously. For teams to succeed at TQ, the teams must be empowered. This means granting them a significant degree of control over processes, including the ability to revise processes in order to improve them. Managers who wish to empower teams must ensure that participants have the necessary training and the tools and resources to accomplish improvements.

As another part of empowerment, managers must establish a climate in which workers feel comfortable participating actively in TQ efforts. A good example of this is found at Abington Memorial Hospital (http://www.amh.org), which received the 2003 American Hospital Association Quest for Quality Prize in recognition of its success in quality improvement efforts. At Abington every new employee, as part of their induction into the organization and as an element of empowerment, signs an agreement with the following statement: "We, as human beings, in our roles as health professionals, will always make mistakes. We cannot change the human condition but we can change the systems within which we work" ("Abington Memorial Wins . . ." 2003, p. 5). The hospital's chief patient safety officer says this step is taken with new employees to help foster a "climate in which it is safe to admit a mistake, as well as to explore why mistakes may occur" ("Abington Memorial Wins . . ." 2003, p. 5).

Determinants of Effective Teams. Managers can do a great deal to support improvement teams. Effective teams achieve two important results: work is accomplished and participants enjoy the experience. Both are important concerns of program and project managers. Figure 7.8 summarizes the factors and the complex interactions that determine a team's effectiveness. As can be seen in this figure, effectiveness results from several factors that managers can influence, including how teams are structured and how teams operate.

A team's structure is most visible in terms of who participates on the team. Determination of a team's *composition* should be guided by answers to two questions. (1) What knowledge or information is required to address a specific problem or issue or to accomplish the general objective of process improvement? (2) Who possesses or can acquire the required knowledge or information? Team members typically come from within the program or project, but in considering team composition, managers may want to include people from outside the program or project. For example, a program organized to receive referrals from local hospitals may find it beneficial to include participants from those organizations as members of improvement teams or as consultants to the teams.

Consideration should also be given to how well potential members can work together in determining the composition of improvement teams. This consideration, however, is secondary to considerations of the knowledge needed and of who has or can obtain knowledge in order to accomplish improvements;

FIGURE 7.8. KEY DETERMINANTS OF TEAM EFFECTIVENESS.

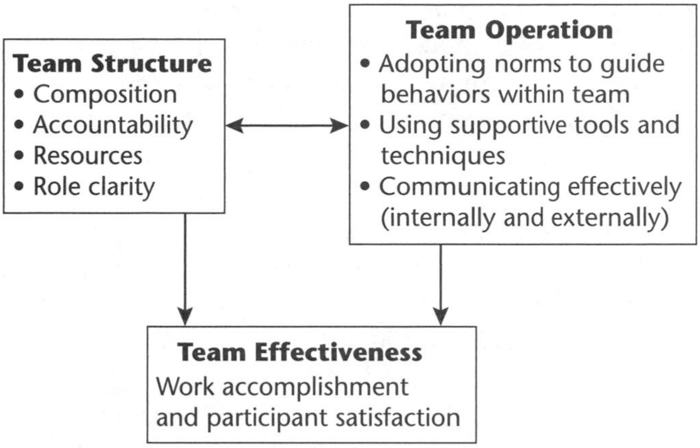

participants' difficulties in working together can usually be overcome by how a team is structured and how a team operates, as is discussed next.

A basic part of a team's structure is the establishment of *accountability* for and within the team. For example, managers can appoint team leaders and imbue them with authority over other participants. Appointed team leaders can also be held responsible for team performance. Alternatively, managers can leave it to teams to select their own leaders or to function under a team-developed plan for rotating the leader role. Experience with improvement teams in many settings has shown that teams are more participative and democratic when managers assign accountability to the team and leave it to participants to negotiate the leader role as well as how the work of the team will be accomplished.

Another important structural consideration is that of the *resources* needed for a team's effectiveness. Resource requirements vary in differing situations, but all improvement teams require resources. Often, no resource is more important than appropriate training in team participation techniques and strategies for participants. Specific training for those who lead or facilitate CI teams in the use of the tools and techniques of CI is vital to the success of improvement teams.

Other resource allocation decisions managers face in structuring improvement teams include financial resources or budget commitments; time for participants to attend team meetings and engage in team activities; and access to information needed to effectively address a problem or identify and make general process improvements. Examples of such informational needs include management reports, clinical data, regulatory requirements, and plans.

Furthermore, as is also shown in Figure 7.8, teams also need *role clarity* if they are to succeed. Managers establish teams to accomplish explicit purposes. The purposes must be specified for a team and any constraints or limits on the team must be clarified at the outset of its work, including required timelines, budgets, or form of communicating results of a team's work. This can be called *chartering* a team. A team charter, which can be provided verbally but is more useful in written form, typically includes information such as the following:

- A brief overview of the process to be improved
- A statement about why the process needs to be improved or considered for improvement
- A proposal for how the team will demonstrate the process has improved
- A timeline for the team's work
- Resources available to the team and constraints on the team
- How and to whom the team should communicate its progress and its final product

Establishing role clarity does not necessarily mean that managers impose all the norms or operational practices (which are discussed next) on a team. A team may have considerable latitude in determining for itself how it will approach resolving a problem or accomplishing an improvement goal. Teams formed for the general purpose of improvement, in fact, may even be free to select the problems or issues they wish to address. However, this and all aspects of a team's role must be clearly established as part of the team structure.

Two especially important roles played within successful teams are *team leader* and *team facilitator*. It is possible, but not necessary, for these roles to be played by a single individual. Both roles are necessary to effective teams because the work of teams has two components, task and process. The task component involves accomplishing the work for which the team is formed—that is, making improvements in processes that enhance quality or other aspects of performance. The process component of a team's work, which is essential for the task component to be accomplished, involves how the team members work together as they interact in performing their tasks. A team's leader can focus on the task component, while its facilitator can focus on the processes of team performance. The leader keeps participants on track toward accomplishing the objectives established for or by the team, while the facilitator monitors participation and interactions and intervenes as necessary to keep things working smoothly.

Improvement teams whose membership compositions have been carefully considered, for which accountability has been clearly established, to which necessary resources have been made available, and whose roles have been clearly defined, are more likely to be effective than teams that do not possess these advantages. However, the structure of teams does not fully explain their effectiveness, either in terms of work accomplishment or participant satisfaction. Effective teams must also operate effectively.

As can be seen in Figure 7.8, team operation requires that teams adopt and use *norms* that can guide individual participant and team behaviors. A norm is a "standard that is shared by team members and regulates member behavior" (Fried, Topping, and Rundall 2000, p. 166). How teams develop norms is largely influenced by how accountabilities for and within teams are established. Operational norms can be imposed or the team itself can determine norms. The latter is usually a better approach.

Norms that support improvement teams' operation include commitment to continuous improvement, attendance expectations, importance of achieving consensus decisions, giving full attention to tasks, being respectful of diverse opinions and views, and accepting responsibility for the teams' success. The most important operational norm for improvement teams is commitment to continuous improvement. This commitment can be buttressed by the fact that participants prefer being associated with programs and projects that are known for providing quality services. Moreover, quality services can be accomplished in part through programs' and projects' commitment to improvement.

A second team operation variable that influences effectiveness is a team's use of supportive improvement *tools and techniques*. Several of these tools were described previously, including benchmarking, workflow charting, cause-and-effect (fishbone) diagrams, Pareto diagrams, and run charts. Other tools and techniques that are useful to improvement teams include such group processes as conflict-resolution and negotiation strategies (LaFasto and Larson 2001).

Improvement teams often benefit from considering themselves problem-solving groups and using a basic problem-solving process model as an integral technique in their work. Figure 7.9 is one such model. The reader should note this problem-solving process model bears a close structural resemblance to the basic decision-making process model shown in Figure 5.2. Both processes follow similar pathways.

A final team operation variable that is crucial to team effectiveness is how well a team communicates, both internally and externally. As defined in Chapter Six, *communicating* effectively means creating or exchanging understanding between senders and receivers. "It is incumbent upon team leaders to manage communications within a team and between the team and external groups" (Fried, Topping, and Rundall 2000, p. 180).

FIGURE 7.9. MODEL OF PROBLEM-SOLVING PROCESS FOR IMPROVEMENT TEAMS.

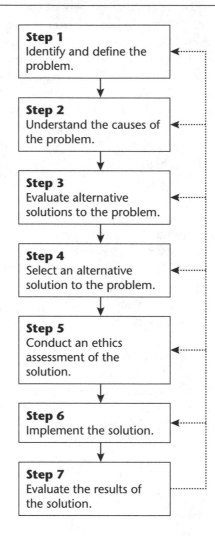

A model of the technical process of communicating is shown in Figure 6.3, including the roles played by contextual and personal barriers that hinder effective communication. You may wish to review that material, paying close attention to the discussion of how the barriers to communication can be overcome.

This is highly relevant to effectively communicating within improvement teams. Information about overcoming barriers to communication is also relevant to communication a team may have about its work with people not directly involved on the team, such as describing the team's results or recommendations.

In many situations, the most important communications in a CI effort occur within the first meeting of the improvement team. This is when a tone and pattern are set for subsequent work, when the team's purposes and accountabilities are established, and when information is provided about how the team will operate. The first meeting of an improvement team should be carefully planned. Planning participants should include the manager who is chartering or establishing the team, the team leader if the person is appointed rather than selected later by the team, and the team facilitator. A typical agenda for a first meeting of an improvement team includes the following:

- Introduce participants (as needed), clarify team leader and facilitator roles, and explain what other team members can contribute to the improvement effort.
- Discuss the team's charter if there is one, or discuss the purpose for which the team has been established.
- Discuss norms (which can be added to later) that will guide the team.
- Discuss the approach the team will take, such as the FOCUS-PDCA model, as well as supportive tools and techniques that will be used.
- Develop a schedule for the team's work, focusing on the next meeting by deciding who will do what and by when.
- Evaluate the meeting by discussing what went well and what did not. This step permits the team to improve as it goes and brings closure to the meeting.

Subsequent meetings can be structured by following steps 3 through 9 of the FOCUS-PDCA model of improvement (see Figure 7.4). These meetings will be more productive if the team leader and team facilitator establish objectives for each meeting and develop and distribute an agenda, including time allocation for each agenda item, prior to the team meetings.

To conclude, as the discussion of the three guiding principles—patient/customer focus, continuous improvement, and teamwork—used by managers as they pursue TQ approaches to quality in their programs and projects suggests, the challenges of managing quality are best met through a systematic approach. Although they may differ in details, successful TQ approaches to managing quality share a number of elements, no matter what the setting in which they occur.

For example, in a review of quality efforts in major American corporations, the U.S. General Accounting Office (1991) identified the following features typical of successful quality improvement initiatives:

- Organizations determine what their customers want and need and have processes in place to meet those needs.
- Managers provide active leadership to establish quality as a fundamental value, which is incorporated into the organization's management philosophy.
- Quality concepts are clearly articulated and thoroughly integrated throughout all activities of the organization.
- Managers establish a corporate culture that involves all employees in contributing to quality improvement.
- Organizations focus on employee involvement, teamwork, and training in quality improvement tools at all levels.
- Total quality management systems are based on a continuous and systematic approach to gathering, evaluating, and acting on facts and data.

These characteristics of TQ approaches in the most successful corporations apply fully to the health programs and projects that succeed at continuously improving the quality of their services.

Summary

This chapter emphasizes that quality is important to those who receive services from health programs and projects, as well as to the participants who work in them. The importance of quality both to those who receive and those who provide a program or project's services is relevant to its manager. Patients/customers want health services to be of high technical quality with appropriate attention paid to their values, their physical and psychological comfort, and their need for open communication with those who provide the services. The importance to participants derives from the fact that those who work in programs and projects that strive to continuously improve quality enjoy higher levels of satisfaction from their work.

This chapter defines quality as it applies to health services as "the degree to which health services for individuals and populations increase the likelihood of desired health outcomes and are consistent with current professional knowledge" (Institute of Medicine 1990, p. 21). The dual components of quality are described as content quality (the clinical expertise and technical aspects of providing health services) and delivery and service quality (the interpersonal aspects of providing health services). Interpersonal aspects include empathy, communication, and being able to meet patients/customers' requirements and expectations for convenience, timeliness, and the like.

Measurement of quality is described in terms developed by Donabedian (1980), who notes that the measurement of quality rests on structural measures (innate characteristics of those who provide services and of the settings in which they are provided); process measures (what service providers do to patients/customers), and outcome measures (what happens to the health of patients/customers as a result of services).

Following a brief review of the evolution of various approaches to managing quality, a systematic approach termed a total quality (TQ) approach is described in detail. This approach to managing quality in programs or projects is guided by three principles: patient/customer focus, continuous improvement, and teamwork. Figure 7.1 illustrates the interconnected nature of these principles.

The patient/customer focus requires that a health program or project identify what its patients/customers need and want, and then design and deliver services that satisfy those needs and wants. Continuous improvement means managers commit to ongoing efforts to examine the processes through which services are provided in search of better ways to provide the services. Teamwork is emphasized because TQ is a collective responsibility of all those involved in a program or project.

FOCUS-PDCA, the most widely used continuous improvement model, is described in detail and shown in Figure 7.4. The FOCUS part of the acronym derives from the following:

Find a process to improve.

Organize an improvement team and necessary resources.

Clarify current knowledge about the process.

Understand the process and sources of variation in it.

Select an improvement or intervention.

The PDCA part of the acronym is based on a model developed by Shewhart intended to guide managers in planning an action to improve a process based on careful study of the process, implementing the action on a small scale, checking to see how it conforms to the plan, and then acting on what is learned as follows:

Plan how to implement the intervention.

Do it by initiating the intervention, often on a small scale at first.

Check the results of the early implementation, revising as necessary until it proves itself as an improvement.

Act on what was learned in the check step. If the change was successful, incorporate it on a larger scale and make it permanent. If not, go through the cycle again with a different plan.

The application of the FOCUS-PDCA model is exemplified in the chapter by describing how a continuous improvement (CI) team, established in a family practice program to improve the care of people with type 2 diabetes, followed the steps in the model as they undertook a successful CI effort.

A number of tools useful in support of CI are described, including: benchmarking, workflow charting, cause-and-effect (fishbone) diagrams, Pareto diagrams, and run charts. A comprehensive model (see Figure 7.8) of the determinants of successful improvement teams is presented, showing that a team's effectiveness results from several aspects of how teams are structured and how they operate.

Chapter Review Questions

1. Define quality as it applies to health programs and projects. Distinguish between (1) content quality and (2) delivery and service quality.
2. Discuss the importance of managing quality in a health program or project.
3. Discuss Donabedian's approach to measuring quality.
4. List and briefly describe the three principles that underpin a total quality (TQ) approach to managing quality in health programs and projects.
5. Discuss the role of continuous improvement (CI) in managing quality.
6. Draw the FOCUS-PDCA model of CI.
7. List and briefly describe several tools useful in CI.
8. Draw a model of the determinants of work team effectiveness.
9. Describe the roles of team leaders and team facilitators in successful CI teams.
10. Write an agenda for a first meeting of a newly formed CI team and describe briefly why each agenda item is important.

CHAPTER EIGHT

COMMERCIAL AND SOCIAL MARKETING

Managers of health programs and projects can use marketing in two important ways as they perform their work. The financial or commercial success of many programs and projects is affected by the use of *commercial marketing*. In addition, especially in programs and projects focused on health promotion and education, *social marketing* is used in the provision of services. Both forms of marketing are defined next and discussed in this chapter

Adapting the most widely cited definition of commercial marketing to the health services context (Kotler and Clarke 1987, p. 5), commercial marketing in health programs and projects is defined as planning, implementing, and evaluating activities designed to bring about voluntary exchanges with people in target markets for the purpose of achieving the desired results established for a program or project.

These exchanges involve things of value to the parties. Obvious target markets of health programs and projects include the existing patients/customers who directly use their products or services, potential new patients/customers who may use their products or services, as well as others who can influence existing or potential patients/customers, such as referring physicians and health plans that may permit or limit use of services by their subscribers or members. Other important target markets are a program or project's potential participants, donors, and volunteers, and in some circumstances an organization in which the program or project is embedded. Commercial marketing focuses on facilitating exchanges between a program or project and its target markets, including identifying and quantifying the target markets.

Adapting a widely used definition of social marketing (Andreasen 1995, p. 7), social marketing in health programs and projects is defined as the application of commercial marketing technologies to planning, implementing, and evaluating services that are designed to influence the voluntary behavior of target audiences in order to improve their personal welfare and that of society. Another useful definition of social marketing is to view it as "a process for influencing human behavior on a large scale, using marketing principles for the purpose of societal benefit rather than commercial profit" (Smith 2000, p. 11).

Thus, both commercial and social marketing can be useful to managers of health programs and projects. After reading the chapter, the reader should be able to do the following:

- Define commercial marketing and understand the basic elements in a commercial marketing strategy for health programs and projects, including the 4 Ps
- Define social marketing and understand the basic elements of using social marketing in health programs and projects
- Understand use of the epidemiological planning model (EPM) in marketing
- Understand the role of evaluation in commercial and marketing strategies

Commercial Marketing Strategies in Health Programs and Projects

Frequently, the success and longevity of programs or the successful completion of projects may depend upon their managers achieving a degree of success in marketing them commercially. This is the case because the central concept of commercial marketing is the establishment and facilitation of voluntary and mutually beneficial exchanges between parties.

The most obvious examples of commercial marketing exchanges involve those between buyers and sellers. The services provided through a program or project, such as a well-baby care or elder care program, may have value to certain people who buy the services either directly or through insurance coverage. When this happens to a sufficient extent, the program or project can be a commercial success. However, many other types of exchanges are also important to programs and projects.

It is essential to attract participants (and volunteers in some situations) to fill the positions in a program or project's organization design. Many programs and projects rely upon donors or grant makers for financial support. It may be necessary to satisfy public and private payers such as Medicaid programs or insurance plans to cover the services provided. Success may depend upon convincing physicians or other health care providers to refer patients to the services. When programs and projects are embedded in larger organizations, it is important to convince the host organization of the value of the program or project in order to sustain its continuation. All of these parties to potential exchanges with a program or project are its target markets and must be addressed through commercial marketing efforts. Thus, the purposes of commercial marketing are broad and can be summarized as building and maintaining exchange relationships with various target markets in order to optimize achievement of the desired results established for a program or project.

Regardless of which target market, or segment or sub-group within a target market, is the focus, the key to commercially marketing a program or project successfully is knowledge of the wants and needs of those in the target markets and segments, coupled with the ability to satisfy some of these wants and needs. To fully appreciate commercial marketing, it is important to understand that it requires identifying wants and needs of those in target markets and being able to fulfill those wants and needs effectively.

Even though establishing and facilitating voluntary and mutually beneficial exchanges between a program or project and its target markets presumes knowledge of the wants and needs of people in the target markets, identifying these wants and needs is not always simple or straightforward. In part, the determination of the wants and needs of patients/customers, donors, participants, or others with whom exchanges may be necessary or desirable is complicated by the fact that people have various types of needs. As a starting point, people have *perceived needs*—that is, what they think they need. Perceived needs become wants, and people often feel very strongly about what they want. For example, certain patients, perhaps influenced by ubiquitous pharmaceutical marketing efforts, may be convinced that they need a specific new drug to address their health problem. The nature of perceived needs varies with individuals. For example, one donor making a significant financial gift to a program or project may want anonymity, while other donors seek widespread publicity about their generosity. These donors have different needs and must be dealt with in different ways if successful exchanges are to occur.

Sometimes, peoples' needs are demonstrated through their decisions and actions. Without knowing what people who enroll in a program actually perceive their needs to be, one might infer merely from a high level of enrollment that the services of a program are needed or wanted. Thus, a second type of need is *expressed need*. This type of need is typically revealed in the numbers of people using particular services.

Especially regarding sophisticated health services, it may be difficult or impossible for people either to perceive their needs or to exhibit expressed needs for the services. They simply do not know of the services or of the benefits they might enjoy through receiving them. Thus, it may be necessary to determine levels of need or want existing in a target market by making judgments about these levels (Hoffman and Bateson 2001). The use of guidelines or norms established through expert opinion is a frequently used means of determining levels of needs and wants in this manner. Determination of what is called *normative need* for health services is routinely based on the opinions of experts about the appropriate (needed) levels of health services for individuals and populations. For example, a panel of public health experts may decide what they believe to be the appropriate levels of certain services to meet the needs for these services in populations of people.

This has been done on a large scale in *Healthy People 2010,* which is a comprehensive set of disease prevention and health promotion objectives for the entire nation. Created by scientists and other experts both inside and outside of government, this document (http://www.healthypeople.gov/Document/tableofcontents.htm.) identifies a wide range of public health priorities and specific, measurable objectives for the health of the nation's population.

On a smaller scale, managers of a program or project may be able to normatively determine need for services in its target market by applying incidence rates that are often available from sources such as the Centers for Disease Control and Prevention (http://www.cdc.gov/nchs/) and from commercial sources such as the MedStat Group (http://www.medstat.com) and Solucient (http://www.solucient.com).

A thorough understanding of the needs of people in a program or project's target markets is the basis for building effective exchange relationships with them. These needs are best understood if perceived, expressed, and normative needs are all taken into account. It is important to determine the needs and wants of people in each of a program or project's target markets, whether patients/customers, potential participants, donors, health professionals who might refer patients/customers, or other relevant target markets. However, for programs and projects that are established to provide services, the potential patients/customers who might use the services are critical target markets and are likely to be the focus of significant commercial marketing efforts.

Identification and quantification of the vital patient/customer target market is described in the next section, followed by a discussion of how this target market is used to develop a commercial marketing strategy to facilitate exchanges with people in a target market. The processes of identifying and quantifying target markets and of designing and implementing marketing strategies to facilitate exchanges with them, however, are similar for all types of target markets.

Identifying and Quantifying Patient/Customer Target Markets

Managers seek to identify and quantify target markets, as well as understand the needs and wants of people in these markets, so they can tailor effective marketing strategies to facilitate exchanges with people in the target markets. To facilitate commercial marketing focused on patient/customer target markets, it may be useful to segment them along any number of dimensions. Examples of patient/customer market segments (or sub-groups) are listed in Table 8.1.

Of course, the identification and quantification of target markets and segments within them is only the beginning of understanding the potential of the target markets and segments to produce actual demand for the services of a program or project. Such determinations require additional analysis, which can be aided by use of techniques such as the epidemiological planning model (Griffith and White 2002). An example of the application of this model follows.

Epidemiological Planning Model. Healthy Start, Inc., a program of the Allegheny County (Pennsylvania) Health Department (http://trfn.clpgh.org/hspgh/index. html), is part of a national demonstration initiative funded by the U.S. Department of Health and Human Services. This program is designed to identify a broad range of community-driven strategies and interventions to reduce infant mortality and the number of low birth-weight babies in communities experiencing high infant mortality rates.

Several of the services provided by Healthy Start are designed for teenage mothers, whose babies are twice as likely to die before their first birthday as babies born to women in their twenties. This program typifies programs in which the level of normative need for services in a target market–which is often one

TABLE 8.1. EXAMPLES OF PATIENT/ CUSTOMER MARKET SEGMENTS.

Type of Market Segment	Shared Group Characteristics
Demographic Segment	Measurable statistics such as age, gender, race, income, occupation, health insurance
Psychographic Segment	Lifestyle preferences such as urban or suburban or rural dwellers, preference for alternative medicine, willingness to use new products or services
Use-Based Segment	Frequency of usage such as medical and dental services, health clubs, fitness centers
Benefit Segment	Desire to obtain certain product or service benefits such as luxury, thriftiness, scheduling convenience, ease of access
Geographic Segment	Location such as zip code, community, region, state

or more demographic categories (such as teenage women) in a geographic community (such as a cluster of zip codes)—can be estimated using the epidemiological planning model (EPM).

The EPM is an equation in the following general form through which an estimate of the demand for a particular service can be made:

$$\left\{\begin{array}{c}\text{Demand for}\\\text{a service}\end{array}\right\} = \left\{\begin{array}{c}\text{Population}\\\text{at risk}\end{array}\right\} \times \left\{\begin{array}{c}\text{Incidence}\\\text{rate}\end{array}\right\} \times \left\{\begin{array}{c}\text{Average use}\\\text{per incidence}\end{array}\right\} \times \left\{\begin{array}{c}\text{Market}\\\text{share}\end{array}\right\}$$

In programs such as Healthy Start, the EPM has many marketing and planning uses. For example, this program's managers may be interested in estimating the demand for counseling services for teenage mothers. An estimate of demand for these services will help ensure the program can provide appropriate services in an effective and timely manner. Effective commercial marketing strategies require that the needs and wants—which translate into demand for services—of those in target markets are known and that programs and projects can effectively satisfy the demands.

The estimate of the demand for counseling services for teenage mothers would be based on current information for terms in the EPM equation, or on projections if managers were interested in projecting demand in future years. In this example, where the service area is Allegheny County, Pennsylvania, the demand calculation for counseling for teenage mothers is made as follows:

- Population at risk is determined from information on the county's population available from the U.S. Census Bureau (http://www.census.gov). There are about 82,000 female teenagers in the county; this statistic can be further broken down into race and age cohorts.
- Incidence rate is determined by using national data on birth rates for teenagers by race and age cohort, available from the National Center for Health Statistics (http://www.cdc.gov/nchs). Overall, the rate is approximately 35 births per 1,000 female teenagers annually. This means there are about 2,870 births to teenage mothers in the county annually ($35 \times 82 = 2,870$).
- Average use of counseling sessions per incident is determined by the number of counseling sessions managers plan to provide to each program client; assume three sessions per client.
- Market share in this situation is based on the fraction of the population at risk that the program's managers think they will serve; this number can be guided by actual experience in an ongoing program. In this instance, assume that 50 percent of the population at risk will be served.

Thus, demand for Healthy Start's counseling services can be *estimated* by the following calculation at 4,305 counseling sessions per year:

$$\begin{Bmatrix} \text{Demand for} \\ \text{counseling} \\ \text{sessions} \end{Bmatrix} = \begin{Bmatrix} \text{Population} \\ \text{at risk} = \\ 82,000 \end{Bmatrix} \times \begin{Bmatrix} \text{Incidence} \\ \text{rate} = \\ 35/1,000 \end{Bmatrix} \times \begin{Bmatrix} \text{Average use} \\ \text{per incidence} = \\ 3 \end{Bmatrix} \times \begin{Bmatrix} \text{Market} \\ \text{share} = \\ 50\% \end{Bmatrix}$$

Once target markets and segments within them are identified and quantified, however, managers still must develop effective commercial marketing strategies; commercial marketing strategies allow them to achieve productive exchanges with the people in target markets and segments. Effective commercial marketing strategies are developed around several interrelated elements. As an applied example, these elements are applied to Healthy Start's efforts to establish effective exchanges with teenage mothers in the following section.

The 4 Ps of a Commercial Marketing Strategy

Successful commercial marketing strategies in any context involve four essential elements: **p**roduct or service, **p**rice, **p**lace, and **p**romotion–the so-called 4 Ps of marketing (Kotler 1982). These four elements of a marketing strategy require concurrent and interactive decisions if desired exchanges with people in target markets are to be accomplished. Figure 8.1 illustrates these relationships. Product (or service), price, place, and promotion each affect the appeal of a program or project's services. The manner in which the 4 Ps are packaged will directly affect the likelihood that the existing and potential patients/customers in a program or project's target markets will enter into the desired exchanges with the program or project.

Product or Service

In the context of health programs and projects, outputs are more often *services* than *products*. Whether a program or project produces services or products, its services or products are critical to successful commercial marketing. From a commercial marketing perspective, a successful product or service is one that satisfies needs and wants of target markets in such a way that those in the target market select the service over alternatives provided by competitors, or over the alternative of not using any service. The challenge is to make the services provided through health programs and projects so attractive and convenient for people in target markets that the services are selected over others that might be available, or in lieu of not using any services. In the example of counseling services for teenage mothers provided by Healthy Start, the services must appeal to people in this specific target market.

FIGURE 8.1. ELEMENTS OF A MARKETING STRATEGY.

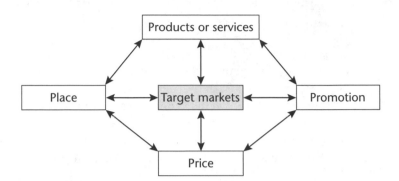

Services often are more difficult to successfully market than products for a variety of reasons, including such characteristics as intangibility, inseparability, perishability, and variability (Ginter, Swayne, and Duncan 2002). Products, such as clothing or computers, are tangible. Products can be picked up, put in a bag, taken home after purchase, and used by the consumer. Services, in contrast, are *intangible*. They are an experience. Production and consumption of services occur simultaneously; consumption is *inseparable* from provision. Provision of health services typically involves repeated episodes of health services providers directly interacting with patients/customers. The fact that production and consumption occur simultaneously means that services cannot be produced in advance and stored for later delivery. The services are in effect *perishable*.

Thus, a key ingredient in successfully marketing service-based programs or projects is a careful matching of the provision of services with the demand for them. It does not matter that services are readily available on weekdays, when people want them on weekends, or that they are available between the hours of 8:00 a.m. and 4:00 p.m., when people prefer them in the evening.

Many variables enter into each service episode: specific service providers vary in terms of ability and attitude; patients/customers vary in terms of needs and expectations; and conditions vary in terms such as how busy a program or project is on a particular day or the availability of support, such as computer systems. These factors typically lead to greater *variability* in the provision of services compared to the tangible products. Services provided through programs and projects are difficult to standardize, and this complicates efforts to commercially market the services.

The most important step that program and project managers can take to ensure services will be attractive and appealing to patients/customers is to base the services on input from people in the target markets identified for the services. This information can be gathered in a variety of ways, including from questionnaires, surveys, or the conduct of focus groups. Information gleaned from patients/customers and potential patients/customers can be used to ensure that services fit their wants and needs.

Other steps that program and project managers can take to make services more attractive and to overcome the challenges inherent in marketing services include the following:

- Select and train staff carefully, including training in effectively interacting with patients/customers in culturally appropriate ways.
- Pay attention to the physical aspects of the service episodes. Décor, ambience, and amenities are important to most people and establish an important dimension of how they view their experience with a program or project.
- Pay attention to the entire process through which exchanges occur with patients/customers. Even if people receive excellent health services that fully address their health problems, they will be concerned about all aspects of their interaction with a program or project. Were they received courteously when they arrived for their appointment? Were they treated with respect, and was their dignity and privacy honored? Did they have to wait past the appointment time? Did they receive a correct bill or was the insurance paperwork properly handled?

Patient/Customer Satisfaction with Services. An important aspect of service performance is patient/customer satisfaction with the services received. Although developed outside the health care context, the SERVQUAL approach to service quality can be useful in guiding efforts to provide services in a manner that satisfies patients/customers of health programs and projects (Parasuraman, Zeithaml, and Berry 1988). This approach identifies five dimensions of service that are important to patients/customers:

Reliability	Providing services dependably and accurately
Assurance	Demonstrating knowledge and courtesy when providing services and also conveying trust and confidence
Responsiveness	Willingness to help and assist patients/customers and to provide services promptly
Empathy	Providing services in a caring and individualized manner to patients/customers
Tangibles	The appearance and amenities of the physical facilities and the appearance and attitudes of those who work in the program or project

Satisfaction levels with the interactions through which patients/customers receive services are determined by both their clinical *and* their service aspects. It is not enough to provide services that are clinically excellent, although this must be done if patients/customers are to be satisfied with services. A broader approach to patient/customer satisfaction acknowledges both clinical and non-clinical aspects of the services a health program or project provides.

A broad approach to patient/customer satisfaction takes into account accessibility and convenience, availability of resources, continuity of care, efficacy and outcomes of care, financial considerations, humaneness, information gathering, information providing, pleasantness of surroundings, and quality and competence of health care personnel (Berkowitz, Pol, and Thomas 1995). All of these variables are relevant in the service element of a commercial marketing strategy. However, no matter how effectively services are designed to satisfy the needs and wants of patients/customers, successful commercial marketing strategies require consideration of additional elements.

Price

The second of the 4 Ps of a commercial marketing strategy is *price*. Even if the services of a program or project respond to the needs of patients/customers in target markets, successful exchanges with the target markets may depend in part upon the price of the service. The most obvious aspect of the price of health services is the dollar amount patients/customers are expected to pay. This is an important aspect of marketing all products and services. However, there is more to price than the monetary value attached to the service. Using services may have other costs such as inconvenience, loss of time, loss of a sense of well-being, or even feelings of indignity.

In regard to many health services, the financial price is not paid directly by patients/customers; at least the price is not fully and exclusively paid by them.

This is the case with the counseling services available to teenage mothers through Healthy Start. Price, except when there are deductibles or co-payment provisions in the coverage, may be of little importance to the direct consumer. In other situations where services are not covered by public or private insurance, then price may be very important to patients/customers, although its importance in their decision making may vary with their personal financial circumstances.

The existence of insurance and public programs frequently affects the role of price in marketing health services, shifting concern about price from patients/customers to those who pay on their behalf. For example, if services are covered by commercial insurance plans, then the price charged to the plans for their subscribers who receive the services are more important to the plans than to the subscribers. Similarly, the prices charged to public payers for services are important to the agencies responsible for reimbursing providers for services.

Price considerations in the decisions people make about consuming services are often weighed in association with *quality* and *utility* considerations. Many people seek services they think are of high quality, of utility to them, and offered at what they consider a fair price. In effect they are seeking *value*.

Considerations of value require that buyers and sellers of services think about not only price, but also quality and utility. In the case of the counseling services provided by Healthy Start, the teenage mothers considering using the services will take into account that the services are available free of charge to them, but they will also weigh such costs as time and inconvenience against their assessment of the benefits they will derive from participating in the counseling sessions. If they do not value the sessions, it will not matter that the direct costs of participation to them is relatively small.

Teenage mothers will also take additional considerations into account as they make decisions about using the counseling services of Healthy Start. The program must also factor these additional considerations into the design of an effective commercial marketing strategy. Even if a program or project has carefully designed its services to meet patients/customers' needs, and has made certain that financial price is not a barrier, other elements must also be considered. For example, the physical location of a program or project can play an important role in its commercial success.

Place

The place where a program or project is physically located can support or hinder its overall success in achieving all its desired results. The teenage mothers to whom Healthy Start wishes to provide counseling services will make their decisions about using the services in part based on where they will receive the services. Invariably, a program or project's accessibility to the people in its target markets influences their decisions about using the program or project's services.

Accessibility is more than physical location. It includes days and hours of operation. The availability of parking and ease of access for people with disabilities are part of the place consideration. Programs that extend weekday hours and remain open on weekends enhance accessibility for many of those who wish to use their services. Similarly, the opening of new locations or the operation of satellite units can enhance access to a program or project's services.

In addition to the importance of physical location, attention must also be given to various aspects of how patients/customers are treated and made to feel upon arrival. Comfortable, attractive, well-lighted reception areas can make them feel welcome. Courteous, respectful, and culturally sensitive reception is an important aspect of a successful place element in a marketing strategy for any program or project.

Luallin and Sullivan (1998) suggest several steps to ensure that a program or project responds to the expectations of those it seeks to serve or attract. First, routinely assess patient/customer-responsive systems and protocols and correct any deficiencies. This assessment should be made in several areas and guided by questions such as the following:

Accessibility	Are office hours convenient for employed patients/customers?
	Are exterior and interior signs attractive and legible?
	Is parking adequate and are provisions made for elderly people and people with disabilities?
	Are all public areas clean and attractive?
Patient/customer flow	Are patients/customers greeted quickly and courteously upon arrival?
	Are those who have contact with patients/customers and other visitors professional, helpful, and friendly?
	Are waiting areas comfortable?
	Are waiting patients/customers kept informed of their situation and seen as quickly as possible?

Patient/customer communication	Are all patients/customers treated as valued clients in all communications?
	Do service providers explain procedures before starting?
	Are educational materials of high quality and readily available?
	Is there an effective way to obtain patient/customer feedback?
	Is patient/customer confidentiality and privacy assured?

The second step in ensuring that a program or project responds effectively to the expectations of those it seeks to serve is to select high-potential participants and train them properly. This step assures that a program or project's staff–including direct service providers and those who support them in this work–contribute positively to the marketing strategy by helping make the place element of the strategy as attractive as possible. Recall from the discussion in Chapter Three that staffing is the process of filling the individual positions established in an organization design for a program or project with appropriate participants.

To be appropriately suited for work in any program or project, individuals must possess relevant technical proficiency in their work, hold the required credentials and certifications, and have experience and training in their roles. In addition, from a marketing strategy perspective, appropriate individuals include those who can relate to patients/customers in a culturally sensitive manner. They must be able to work with people in highly stressful conditions and be able to respond to their needs under such circumstances.

Program and project managers can support this step by establishing performance standards and expectations that go beyond the procedural aspects of work and extend to the service aspects. Luallin and Sullivan (1998, p. 293) recommend the use of patient/customer-centered performance standards in the following areas:

- Telephone procedures–making clear that patients/customers are entitled to prompt, courteous telephone communication. This includes requiring such actions as: answering telephone promptly and speaking in a friendly, helpful tone of voice; and, when putting callers on hold, asking, "Will you hold, please?" When you return to the line, thank callers for holding.

- Patient/customer handling—making clear that patients/customers are to be greeted and treated with respect and dignity, and requiring such actions as: (1) greeting patients/customers and other visitors promptly and establishing eye contact with them; (2) looking for ways to reassure anxious patients/customers; (3) concluding every patient/customer encounter with a "thank you" for the opportunity to provide services.
- Communicating with patients/customers—making clear they are to receive prompt, courteous, and accurate responses to their questions and concerns, and requiring such actions as: (1) making certain the information given to patients/customers is accurate; (2) explaining procedures carefully and asking if there are questions before proceeding; (3) telling patients/customers what you plan to do and not making promises that cannot be kept; (4) following through on all promises made to patients/customers; (5) solving patient/customer's problems as responsively as possible.
- Professional standards—making clear that patients/customers will be assured of high quality care and services, delivered professionally, and requiring such actions as: following dress codes, wearing name badges correctly, and being courteous to patients/customers and other program or project staff.

The standards and actions noted previously must be tailored to specific circumstances and settings, but they provide a template for adding a service focus to what is expected of participants who work in any program or project. In order for the standards to have their full impact, it is necessary for managers to recognize performance that meets the standards, including merit pay increases that reflect service performance as well as the technical competence displayed in work.

As Healthy Start's managers consider a commercial marketing strategy to encourage and facilitate mutually beneficial exchanges with teenage mothers, in addition to carefully designing services to meet teenage mothers' needs (by, for example, addressing any price issues and making the place where services will be received appealing and convenient), the managers must address a fourth element in their strategy, promotion (see Figure 8.1).

Promotion

The fourth P in a commercial marketing strategy is *promotion*. Through promotion, a program or project's manager seeks to establish and maintain its reputation or image, inform patients/customers and their intermediaries about the types and quality of services offered, and provide information about accessing the services.

A program or project with multiple target markets is likely to have different images with each of them. For example, patients/customers may see it as a convenient source of health services of a particular type. Present and potential participants may see it as a good place to work. Referring physicians may see it as a good place to send patients because of the high quality of the services. Insurance plans may see it as practicing better than average utilization control. Competitors may see the program or project as a threat to their own success. The general public may have an image of the program or project as a potential source of particular services should they ever need them.

Typically, health programs and projects seek to establish effective levels of familiarity and perceived attractiveness with target markets through such promotional activities as issuing annual reports, maintaining informative Web sites, publishing newsletters and brochures, and having participants give public lectures on topics related to the program or project. At the extreme, promotion may include purchased media exposure, support or sponsorship of local athletic or social events, and distribution of items such as coffee mugs or t-shirts bearing the name and logo of the program or project.

Well-designed brochures can be among a program or project manager's best tools for promotion. They are sometimes called *identity and capabilities brochures,* which denotes their basic uses: providing enough information about the program or project for readers to identify it—and providing descriptions that inform readers about the program or project's capabilities and services. In some instances, a brochure may also contain information that supports access to and use of the services provided. For example, a section of the brochure can contain a map and parking information, as well as contact information, information about referral arrangements, and payment and billing practices.

Although brochures tend to be idiosyncratic to programs and projects, effective ones include the following types of information:

- Welcome and Introduction—This section should reflect the program or project's appreciation for being selected as a service provider and should include a statement of desire to warrant and maintain patients/customers' trust.
- Mission Statement—This section contains the mission statement and vision for the program or project. It might also include a brief history and important affiliations.
- Services and Capabilities—This section describes in easily understood terminology the specific services available through the program or project, as well as special capabilities. For example, if the program provides counseling services, these may be described along with special capabilities in communicating in various languages. (In fact, depending upon the target market demographics, it might be necessary to provide brochures in more than one language.)

- Operating Policies and Practices–This section, which is optional but often needed, contains practical information such as how to schedule an appointment, billing and payment options, and insurance form processing.
- Staff–This section contains information about the program or project's key professional participants. Depending upon the number of people involved, this might be in the form of a list with information about how to obtain additional information from a Web site or directory. If space permits, brief biographies of key professional participants can be included in the brochure.

The media provides several opportunities for programs and projects to be effectively promoted. The following activities are useful means through which managers can use the media in promotional efforts:

- Developing and distributing to local media press kits that contain detailed information about programs and projects, including awards and measures of performance, along with photographs and information about specific services. The kits can include contact information for satisfied patients/customers who might be interviewed if this has been cleared with them beforehand.
- Issuing press releases to alert the press to major events such as prizes or awards, large grants, or achievement of accreditation. Including information that explains who, what, where, why, and when–and perhaps photographs and quotes–helps reporters do their jobs and enhances the chances they will develop the material into a story.
- Producing public service announcements (PSAs) to reach target markets through television and radio stations. In many communities, radio stations and some television stations provide public service announcements free of charge for nonprofit programs and projects. Of course the production costs must be covered, but sometimes assistance with this can be obtained on a pro bono basis from production companies.
- Writing informative articles for local newspapers and magazines reflecting *technical expertise* about health issues, and describing what programs or projects are doing to address the issues, promotes authors as well as the programs or projects with which they are affiliated.
- Writing editorials and letters to the editor for local newspapers and magazines, especially if they present balanced viewpoints in brief essays of about 300–900 words, can be an effective means of promotion.

Some programs or projects benefit from the assistance of others in their promotion. For example, the Healthy Start program in Allegheny County benefits from the fact that similar programs established in communities across the United

States have formed an association, the National Healthy Start Association (http://www.healthystartassoc.org). The mission of this association is to promote Healthy Start programs through a wide range of activities and efforts that are rooted in the communities the programs serve and actively involve the programs' target markets in their design and implementation.

In some instances, as is the case with Healthy Start, image building reaches the level of *branding*. In addition to programs that are associated with widespread initiatives such as Healthy Start, other programs or projects may benefit from the promotional efforts of the organizations in which they are embedded when the home organization is branded. For example, the Bone Health Program of Magee-Womens Hospital (http://www.magee.edu) in Pittsburgh benefits from the association with the hospital's branding efforts. Because the hospital is part of a large integrated health system, both the program and the hospital also benefit from the system's branding efforts.

When target markets or segments are accurately identified and quantified, when the needs and wants (translated into demand) of the people in the target markets or segments are understood, and when commercial marketing strategies are appropriately developed and implemented by integrating the 4 Ps of product or service, price, promotion, and place, then commercial marketing can serve a program or project well. These activities will help encourage and facilitate mutually beneficial exchanges between programs and projects and their vital patients/customers. Successful commercial marketing strategies will also encourage and facilitate mutually beneficial exchanges with participants, donors, and volunteers—as well as strengthen the support of organizations in which programs and projects are embedded, and improve relationships with regulatory agencies and grant makers.

As noted at the beginning of this chapter, two types of marketing are important to health programs and projects. In addition to commercial marketing strategies discussed previously, some programs and projects use social marketing as a key tool in the services they provide.

Social Marketing in Health Programs and Projects

Social marketing was defined earlier in this chapter as a process of using elements of commercial marketing to influence the voluntary behavior of individuals and groups of people for their own benefit and, in some instances, for the larger society's benefit. The expression "social marketing" was first used in 1971 when Kotler and Zaltman defined it as "the design, implementation, and control of programs calculated to influence the acceptability of social ideas" (Kotler and Zaltman 1971, p. 4).

Health Canada, which is the federal department responsible for helping the people of Canada maintain and improve their health, points out that social marketing is in essence "a new way of thinking about some very old human endeavors. As long as there have been social systems, there have been attempts to inform, persuade, influence, motivate, to gain acceptance for new adherents to certain sets of ideas, to promote causes and to win over particular groups, to reinforce behavior or to change it—whether by favor, argument or force" (Health Canada, Social Marketing Network Web site, http://www.hc-sc.gc.ca/english/socialmarketing). In recent decades, social marketing has been used widely in areas such as energy conservation, recycling, and especially in addressing health issues.

In the United States, social marketing has been used to address such health issues as anti-smoking, safety, drug abuse, drinking and driving, HIV and AIDS, nutrition, physical activity, immunization, breast cancer screening, mental health, family planning, and many other issues. Canada, especially, has made significant use of social marketing in seeking to improve the health of Canadians through widespread social marketing campaigns.

Health Canada has created a Marketing and Creative Services Division and charged it with helping individuals make positive impacts on their own health, the health and well-being of their friends and family, and, ultimately, of the larger society. The division makes extensive use of social marketing in pursuing its goals and maintains a Web site (http://www.hc-sc.gc.ca/english/socialmarketing/social_marketing/tutorial/index.html) containing very helpful information on social marketing, including a seven-step tutorial on developing a social marketing plan.

There are other models and frameworks for using social marketing in health programs and projects. One of the most widely used is the Social Marketing Assessment and Response Tool (SMART), which contains the interactive phases of activities shown in Figure 8.2.

Key Elements in a Social Marketing Strategy

Managers can enhance the success of their social marketing initiatives by taking a *systematic* approach to developing and implementing social marketing strategies (Kotler, Roberto, and Lee 2002). Lagarde (1998) describes the key elements of effective social marketing strategies by suggesting these strategies work best when those who are designing and implementing the strategies do the following:

- Adopt a patient/customer-centered orientation, rather than simply focusing on the message to be conveyed. Conducting formative research, which may be as simple as assuring that the people in the target markets can read and understand the message, supports this orientation. This orientation requires that

FIGURE 8.2. PHASES OF THE SOCIAL MARKETING ASSESSMENT AND RESPONSE TOOL (SMART).

Phase I	Preliminary Planning for Social Marketing Intervention • Identify the health issue or problem of focus • Develop goals for interventions • Outline preliminary plans for evaluation of interventions
Phase II	Patient/Customer Analysis • Identify target markets and segment them • Determine patient/customer needs and wants • Develop preliminary ideas for interventions
Phase III	Social Marketing Strategy • Establish plans for 4 Ps (product/service, price, place, and promotion) • Identify partners, competitors, and allies • Identify individual and societal exchange goods, benefits, values
Phase IV	Develop Interventions • Design interventions based on patient/customer analysis and social marketing strategy • Communicate with partners and clarify roles • Pretest and refine the interventions
Phase V	Implement Social Marketing Strategy • Activate the interventions • Document the process and compare to goals and plans • Continually refine the interventions
Phase VI	Evaluate Social Marketing Strategy • Assess the degree to which target markets are receiving the interventions • Ensure that interventions are consistent with plans and protocols; refine interventions as necessary • Analyze changes in the target markets

Source: Adapted from Rosemary Thackery, and Brad L. Neiger, "Use of Social Marketing to Develop Culturally Innovative Diabetes Interventions," *Diabetes Spectrum,* Vol. 16, No. 1 (January 2003): 15–20. Copyright © 2003 American Diabetes Association. Adapted with permission from the American Diabetes Association.

representatives of target markets be actively involved as the social marketing strategy is initially developed so that it fits their needs, wants, perceptions, lifestyles, media habits, and other attributes. The use of focus groups made up of representatives of target markets can be especially useful in assuring a patient/customer focus.

- Carefully segment target markets. Segmentation based on predisposition, motives, values and lifestyle is essential when designing social marketing strategies. For example, social marketing about exercise will be different for teenagers and the elderly.
- Take into account real and perceived barriers (things that prevent people from adopting a new behavior) facing target markets. Taking barriers into account means being willing to modify interventions to surmount the barriers, including taking action to address the systems or structures that create the barriers. For example, part of an anti-smoking strategy might involve taking steps to ensure that anti-smoking regulations are enforced.
- Demonstrate the benefits of desired change for people in the target markets by showing how their needs and interests are served. This requires recognizing that the needs and wants of people in target markets may differ from those ascribed to them by public health professionals and other program or project participants and can only be determined by analysis of the target markets.
- Use a variety of means or channels to reach target markets through the media, face-to-face communication, and planned and structured events. The methods selected should be based on analysis of the target markets.
- Pre-test the interventions and monitor and evaluate them as the strategy is implemented. Modify the interventions as necessary based on the results of ongoing evaluation (see the discussion of evaluation in a subsequent section of this chapter).
- Form partnerships that enhance credibility and facilitate access to target markets. Partnerships also may help mobilize the human and financial resources necessary to implement a social marketing strategy.
- Create synergy and complementarity with other approaches to social change. Social marketing strategies alone are rarely sufficient to bring about and sustain change. These strategies sometimes work best when related public policies are enacted. For example, laws requiring the use of seat belts or helmets for motorcyclists strengthen efforts to encourage their use in target markets through social marketing strategies.
- Make a long-term commitment to the strategy. The types of changes that most social marketing strategies seek to create take years and decades rather than weeks or months to accomplish. Commitment also often entails sustained financial support for the strategy.

As has been discussed previously, both commercial and social marketing strategies can play roles in the success of health programs and projects. Effective commercial marketing strategies can help managers identify, quantify, and understand the needs and wants of people in their target markets, whether patients/customers or other participants who can contribute to the success of their programs and projects. In turn, by effectively packaging the 4 Ps (products and services, prices, places, and promotions) through the design of their marketing strategies, managers can facilitate mutually beneficial exchanges with people in their target markets.

In addition to the usefulness of commercial marketing, many programs and projects also find social marketing strategies useful in achieving their desired results. This is especially so when the program or project's work involves health promotion and education in efforts intended to change behaviors of individuals and groups.

Whether using commercial or social marketing strategies, managers should pay careful attention to the ethics issues that can arise in the use of these strategies. A second important aspect of using either commercial or marketing strategies is the benefit of carefully evaluating the results of these strategies. The ethics and evaluation aspects of marketing strategies are considered in the following sections.

Ethics in Commercial and Social Marketing Strategies

Ethics considerations and issues routinely emerge in the provision of clinical health services and in the overall management of health programs and projects, including in the development and implementation of both commercial and social marketing strategies (Andreasen 2001). Before proceeding, the reader may find it useful to review the section on ethical management of programs and projects in Chapter One, where it was noted that managers can be guided by the application of four key ethics principles: respect for persons, justice, beneficence, and nonmaleficence.

These principles may seem abstract, but they can be very useful guides for those seeking to take an ethical approach in marketing efforts. For example, the principles can be seen implicitly in the six aims for general improvement in health care in the Institute of Medicine's Committee on Quality of Health Care in America when they recommend that health care should be the following:

Safe–avoiding injuries to patients from the care that is intended to help them [*especially reflects the principles of respect for persons and nonmaleficence*]

Effective—providing services based on scientific knowledge to all who could benefit, and refraining from providing services to those not likely to benefit (avoiding underuse and overuse, respectively) [*reflects the principles of respect for persons, justice, beneficence, and nonmaleficence*]

Patient-centered—providing care that is respectful of and responsive to individual patient preferences, needs, and values and ensuring that patient values guide all clinical decisions [*reflects the principles of respect for persons and beneficence*]

Timely—reducing waits and sometimes harmful delays for both those who receive and those who give care [*especially reflects the principles of respect for persons and nonmaleficence*]

Efficient—avoiding waste, including waste of equipment, supplies, ideas, and energy [*especially reflects the principles of respect for persons and nonmaleficence*]

Equitable—providing care that does not vary in quality because of personal characteristics such as gender, ethnicity, geographic location, and socioeconomic status [*especially reflects the principle of justice*] (Institute of Medicine, Committee on Quality of Health Care in America 2001, pp. 39–40)

Kass (2001) suggests a framework for considering the ethical aspects of health interventions, which readily applies to interventions that use social marketing. She suggests that conducting a careful *ethics analysis* increases the likelihood that those who are planning interventions will be meticulous in their reasoning and will be more likely to design interventions based on science and facts and not merely beliefs. Using a health education–based cardiac risk reduction intervention as an example, the steps in conducting an ethics analysis for this intervention are as follows:

Step 1. Determine the desired results of the intervention. The starting point in an ethics analysis of a health intervention is the desired results of the intervention, expressed in terms of health improvements such as reduction of morbidity or mortality. Using the cardiac risk reduction intervention as an example, those who are planning this health education intervention in a target population would establish the desired *impact* of reducing heart attacks in individuals in the target population. This impact would be predicated on desired *outputs,* such as producing and distributing certain educational information about cardiac risk to people in the target population, and on desired *outcomes,* such as individuals in the target population learning relevant facts about cardiac risk and changing their risk-related behavior.

Step 2. Assess the potential effectiveness of the planned intervention in relation to achieving desired outputs, outcomes, and impact. In this step, those planning the intervention would consider the question of how the intervention will achieve the desired results. All interventions have a hypothesis embedded in them, even if the hypothesis is only implicit. Those planning an intervention hypothesize that if we do a, b, and c, then the result will be x, y, and z. For example, the hypothesis upon which the cardiac risk reduction intervention rests is that if individuals in the target population are exposed to risk-reduction information, then they will change their behavior (for example, stop smoking, modify diets, increase exercise) in ways suggested by the information provided; the changes in behavior will result in fewer heart attacks for those in the target population. The planners of this intervention should challenge the assumptions in their hypothesis by examining existing data and evidence about the effectiveness of such interventions. Only if it is reasonably likely that a planned intervention will achieve the desired results established for it should the intervention be implemented.

Step 3. Determine and minimize the known or potential burdens of the planned intervention. Interventions can impose a variety of potential burdens or harms, ranging from physical harm to issues of privacy and confidentiality. Among the various types of interventions, health education interventions tend to impose relatively few burdens. Education-based interventions are voluntary and seek to empower people in the target population with information that equips them to make their own choices and decisions regarding their health. Even though the burdens and potential harms in the planned health education–based cardiac risk reduction intervention may be relatively minor, the known and potential burdens must be determined so they can be minimized.

Once identified, the known and potential burdens of the intervention must be reduced to the lowest possible level. For example, health education interventions are potentially paternalistic when they emphasize changes in behavior. Paternalism is inconsistent with the ethics principle of respect for persons in terms of treating people as autonomous beings. Similarly, education-based interventions can stereotype the target populations if care is not exercised. For example, decisions about who is pictured in educational materials should be carefully considered. If only obese people are pictured, the incorrect message that obesity is the only relevant risk factor may be conveyed.

Step 4. Assure that the intervention is implemented fairly. This step is based upon the principle of justice, which requires that the benefits and the burdens of an intervention be distributed fairly among those affected. For example, unless the cardiac risk reduction intervention is being planned for a specific group within the target population (for example women, the elderly, African American males), perhaps because they have been identified as being at particularly high risk, the intervention should be designed to benefit all members of the target population. Similarly, the intervention should be readily and conveniently available to the entire target population.

Evaluating Commercial and Social Marketing Strategies

Knowing how commercial or social marketing strategies have worked in reaching and influencing target markets is an important step in using marketing effectively and in improving future marketing efforts. Managers must answer such questions as: Did our message reach the intended target markets? Did they believe and accept our message? Ultimately, did they respond as we had hoped? Answers to such questions require that marketing strategies be evaluated.

Three types of evaluations can be conducted on commercial and social marketing strategies, each serving a different purpose. A *formative evaluation* is undertaken to assist those who are responsible for developing a marketing strategy to determine how people in the target markets will react to messages and materials as the messages and materials are being developed. A formative evaluation is conducted as the marketing strategy is being developed. It entails testing the messages and means of distributing them to ensure that target audiences will understand the information communicated through a marketing effort.

A second type of evaluation, *process evaluation,* is used to track how effectively the message reached the target markets. It involves tracking when, where, and how often messages were delivered, as well as how often those in the target markets actually saw or heard the messages.

A third type of evaluation, *outcome evaluation,* focuses on what happened with people in the target markets as a result of the marketing effort. Outcome evaluations can be short-term or long-term. Table 8.2 illustrates the three types of evaluations that can be conducted for both commercial and social marketing strategies.

Typically, health programs and projects do not allocate large shares of their financial resources to evaluating marketing efforts, choosing instead to spend the money on the actual marketing strategy. However, evaluating these efforts is important and can be undertaken with minimal or modest expenditures, as shown in Table 8.2. By learning what works and does not work in marketing efforts, managers can make better use of future marketing expenditures, whether they are for the purpose of improving the commercial success of a program or project or enhancing the likelihood that the use of social marketing strategies will result in desired outputs, outcomes, and impact.

TABLE 8.2. OPTIONS FOR EVALUATING COMMERCIAL OR SOCIAL MARKETING STRATEGIES.

Type of Evaluation	Minimal Resources	Modest Resources	Substantial Resources
Formative	• Focus groups to determine service location and scheduling preferences (commercial) • Readability test of educational material (social)	• Limited survey to determine program or project name recognition (commercial) • Intercept interviews to determine target market attitudes about health behaviors (social)	• Extensive market research designed to segment target markets (commercial) • Extensive health needs assessment for target markets (social)
Process	• Record keeping to track how messages were delivered and received by target markets (commercial and social)	• Checklist review of implementation milestones (commercial and social)	• Conducting complete management audit of implementation, including review by external experts
Outcome, Short-Term	• Tracking changes in use of services such as visits or screenings (commercial) • Tracking adherence, attendance, or compliance with intervention by target markets (social)	• Analyzing changes in referral patterns (commercial) • Monitoring percentage of target markets aware of or participating in intervention (social)	• Calculating changes in share of target markets (commercial) • Assessing target markets for knowledge change through pre- and post-tests of change (social)
Outcome, Long-Term	• Monitoring trends in media coverage (commercial) • Monitoring trends in grant support for an intervention (social)	• Conducting public surveys to determine opinions about program or project (commercial) • Conducting telephone surveys of target markets to determine changes in health behaviors (social)	• Conducting complete review of program or project performance at five-year interval, including audited financial performance (commercial) • Conducting formal studies of changes in health status of target markets (social)

Summary

This chapter addresses two types of marketing that are of use to program and project managers. *Commercial marketing,* which is important to all health programs and projects, is defined as planning, implementing, and evaluating activities designed to bring about voluntary exchanges with people in target markets for the purpose of achieving the program or project's desired results. *Social marketing,* which is useful in many health programs and projects, is defined as the application of commercial marketing technologies to planning, implementing, and evaluating services that are designed to influence the voluntary behavior of target audiences in order to improve their personal welfare and that of society.

Discussion includes how managers identify and quantify target markets and seek to understand the needs and wants of people in these markets. Commercial marketing strategies are considered as a basis for building effective exchange relationships with people in target markets. The importance of understanding the perceived, expressed, and normative needs of people in target markets and market segments is emphasized.

The epidemiological planning model (EPM), which is useful in estimating the size and scope of markets for the services provided by many programs and projects, is described, along with an applied example. It is noted, however, that even after people in target markets and in segments within the markets are identified, quantified, and understood, managers must develop commercial marketing strategies to facilitate exchanges with the people in the targets and segments.

Successful commercial marketing strategies involve four interrelated elements: product or service, price, place, and promotion. Commonly referred to as the 4 Ps of marketing, these elements of a commercial marketing strategy (see Figure 8.1) are the building blocks of successful commercial marketing strategies. The application of each of the four elements to commercial marketing of health programs and projects is discussed.

When effectively managed, commercial marketing strategies will help attract patients/customers directly and through referrals and can help attract participants, donors, and volunteers, as well as the support of organizations in which programs and projects are embedded. Commercial marketing strategies can also improve relationships with regulatory agencies and grant-making organizations.

Social marketing has been used to address such health issues as antismoking, safety, drug abuse, drinking and driving, HIV and AIDS, nutrition, physical activity, immunization, breast cancer screening, mental health, family planning, and many other health issues. Many programs and projects find it integral to their work.

Key components of a systematic approach to social marketing strategies are described and discussed. They include the following:

- Taking a patient/customer-centered orientation
- Segmenting target markets
- Taking into account real and perceived barriers that prevent people in target markets from adopting a new behavior
- Demonstrating the benefits of desired change for people in the target markets
- Using a variety of means or channels to reach target markets
- Pre-testing interventions and monitoring them as the strategy is implemented
- Forming partnerships that enhance credibility and facilitate access to target markets
- Creating synergy and complementarity with other approaches to social change
- Making a long-term commitment to the social marketing strategy

It is noted that ethics considerations routinely arise in the development and implementation of both commercial and social marketing strategies, and that managers must pay attention to how these issues are addressed. They can be guided in these efforts by the application of four key ethics principles: respect for persons, justice, beneficence, and nonmaleficence.

The chapter concludes with a discussion of the role of evaluation in both commercial and social marketing strategies. Three types of evaluations of marketing strategies are described (see Table 8.2). Formative evaluations assist those who are responsible for developing a marketing strategy to determine how people in the target markets will react to messages and materials as they are being developed. Process evaluations permit managers to track how effectively messages reach the people in target markets. Outcome evaluations focus on what happened with people in the target markets as a result of the marketing strategy.

Chapter Review Questions

1. Define commercial marketing and social marketing as they apply to health programs and projects. Why are both important to health programs and projects?
2. Discuss the importance of identifying target markets and segments as the basis for effective commercial marketing strategies.
3. Discuss the usefulness of the epidemiological planning model (EPM) in marketing strategies.
4. Briefly describe the 4 Ps of a commercial marketing strategy.
5. List and describe the five dimensions of service that are important to patients/customers in the SERVQUAL approach to service quality.

6. Write an outline of the topics that should be covered in an identity and capabilities brochure for a program.

7. Describe ways that a program or project can use the media in promotional efforts.

8. Discuss the key components of an effective social marketing strategy.

9. Discuss how managers can avoid ethics problems in developing and implementing commercial and social marketing strategies.

10. Briefly describe three types of evaluations that can be done on commercial and social marketing strategies. Give an example of the use of each by a program or project manager.

EPILOGUE

The purpose of this epilogue is to recapitulate and emphasize two key aspects of managing health programs and projects. First, although programs and projects vary in many ways, all can be usefully thought of in terms of their logic models; understanding a program or project's logic model reveals much about any program or project. Second, although managing health programs and projects has been discussed in terms of the separate core and facilitative activities managers engage in as they manage, it is necessary to consider the entire set of activities and their inter-connectedness, if the nature of management work is to be understood.

The template for a program or project's logic model is reproduced as Figure E.1. We discuss how a manager establishes the desired results for a program or project, expressing them in terms of outputs, outcomes, and impact. The desired results established for a program or project are an integral component of its logic model, driving much about the design of other components of the model. The manager must carefully consider the processes through which inputs/resources are used to produce the program or project's desired results.

In designing the inputs/resources component of a program or project's logic model, the manager focuses on the human, financial, technological, and organizational inputs necessary to achieve the established desired results. Each program or project is likely to require a unique package of inputs/resources, typically

FIGURE E.1. THE LOGIC MODEL OF A PROGRAM OR PROJECT.

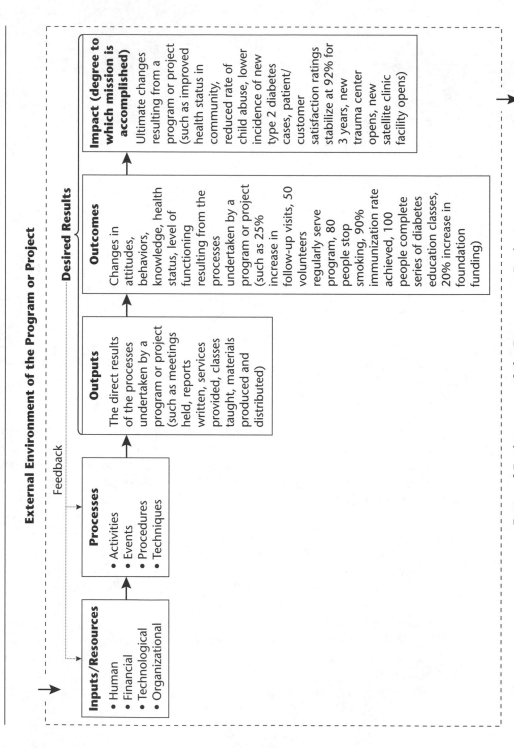

including some mix of resources in the form of paid staff and volunteers, funding, collaborators, technologies, organizational arrangements, physical facilities, equipment, and supplies.

In designing the processes component of a program or project's logic model, the manager focuses on activities, events, procedures, and techniques necessary to use the inputs/resources to accomplish the established desired results. Because each program or project is unique in some ways, including in the desired results established for it, each requires a particular set of processes to achieve the desired results. Determining the desired results for a program or project and then designing the inputs/resources and processes necessary to achieve the desired results is a complicated undertaking. This challenge is magnified by the fact that logic models are not static; they undergo continuing revision throughout the life of a program or project.

Program or project management has been defined in this book as the activities through which the desired outputs, outcomes, and impact of a program or project are established and pursued through various processes using human and other resources. Thus, in performing management work, managers do the following:

- Determine a program or project's desired outputs, outcomes, and impact
- Assemble the necessary inputs and resources to achieve the desired results
- Determine the processes necessary to accomplish the desired results and ensure processes are carried out effectively and efficiently
- Analyze variables in the program or project's external environment, assess their importance and relevance, and respond to them appropriately

In performing management work, the manager engages in an interrelated set of core activities (strategizing, designing, and leading) and facilitative activities (decision making, communicating, managing quality, and marketing). Figure 1.4 was initially presented as a means of illustrating the integrated and intertwined nature of these core and facilitative activities. Now that the activities have been discussed separately and in depth, it is important to reemphasize their interconnectedness. To understand managing, it is necessary to understand the entire, intertwined set of activities depicted in Figure 1.4, here reproduced as Figure E.2. Each component in Figure E.2 affects and is affected by every other component.

As a manager performs the strategizing activity, he lays the foundation to guide designing the remainder of the program or project's logic model and its organization design. The desired results established through strategizing the future of a program or project also guide the manager's leading of the other participants in the program or project. The core activities of managing are closely and fully interrelated. No one activity can be performed well in isolation from

FIGURE E.2. THE CORE AND FACILITATIVE ACTIVITIES IN MANAGEMENT WORK.

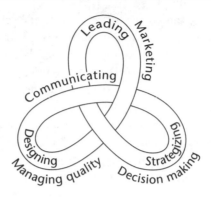

the others, and how well a manager performs any one of the core activities affects performance of the others.

A program or project's manager constantly engages in decision making. This facilitative activity permeates all other activities of managing. In strategizing the future of a program or project, its manager decides about desired results and how to accomplish them. Myriad decisions are made as the manager establishes and revises the program or project's logic model and organization design. The manager must decide how to encourage and facilitate the contributions of other participants as they lead the program or project. Similarly, decisions are made about how and with whom to communicate, how to approach managing quality, and how to design and implement marketing strategies for the program or project.

Like decision making, communicating pervades all other management activities. When managers interact with other participants in strategizing the future of a program or project, they must communicate. Managers also communicate when developing and revising a program or project's logic model and organization design. In leading other participants, managers must communicate with them about their needs and about how these needs can be partially met in the workplace. Communication is essential to efforts to manage quality and is the essence of implementing both commercial and social marketing strategies.

Managing quality in a program or project is directly affected by how well a manager performs the other activities of managing. Conversely, effectively managing quality in a program or project means continuously improving all aspects of its performance. Finally, in thinking about the inter-connectedness of the activities shown in Figure E.2, marketing the services of a well-managed program or project is much easier, all else being equal, than marketing the services of a poorly managed counterpart, simply because there is a direct connection between how well a program or project's managers perform and the quality, value, and appropriateness of the services.

Indeed, the activities of management work form a complex and challenging mosaic. Those who are, or who would be, managers can see that success in any of the core and facilitative activities of management work enhances the likelihood for success in each and all of the other activities. Similarly, inattention to or ineptitude in the performance of any of the activities diminishes performance of each of the other activities and of the whole they comprise. The key to managing health programs and projects successfully that is to having a good logic model and making it work well—is to perform the challenging activities of management work well. I hope this book contributes to the reader's ability to successfully manage health programs and projects.

REFERENCES

"Abington Memorial Wins the 2003 Quest for Quality Prize," *AHA News,* Vol. 39, No. 16 (August 11, 2003): 5.

Abrams, Rhonda. *The Successful Business Plan: Secrets and Strategies.* Palo Alto, Calif.: Running R Media, 2000.

Adams, J. Stacy. "Toward an Understanding of Inequity," *Journal of Abnormal and Social Psychology* 67 (November 1963): 422–436.

Adams, J. Stacy. "Inequity in Social Exchanges," in *Advances in Experimental Social Psychology.* Vol. 2., ed. Leonard Berkowitz. New York: Academic Press, 1965.

Alderfer, Clayton P. "A New Theory of Human Needs," *Organizational Behavior and Human Performance* 4 (May 1969): 142–175.

Alderfer, Clayton P. *Existence, Relatedness, and Growth: Human Needs in Organizational Settings.* New York: Free Press, 1972.

American College of Healthcare Executives, *Healthcare Executive,* (Vol. 18, No. 6): 52–53.

American Organization of Nurse Executives. *Market-Driven Nursing: Developing and Marketing Patient Care Services.* San Francisco: Jossey-Bass, 1999.

Andreasen, Alan R. *Marketing Social Change: Changing Behavior to Promote Health, Social Development, and the Environment.* San Francisco: Jossey-Bass, 1995.

Andreasen, Alan R. *Ethics in Social Marketing.* Washington, D.C.: Georgetown University Press, 2001.

Ashmos, Donde P. "Building Effective Health Care Teams," in *Handbook of Health Care Management,* eds. W. Jack Duncan, Peter M. Ginter, and Linda E. Swayne. Malden, Mass.: Blackwell Publishers (1998): 313–338.

Atkinson, John W. *An Introduction to Motivation.* New York: Van Nostrand, 1961.

Atkinson, John W., and Joel O. Raynor. *Motivation and Achievement.* Washington, D.C.: Winston, 1974.

Austin, Charles J., and Stuart Boxerman. *Quantitative Analysis for Health Services Administration.* Chicago: Health Administration Press, 1995.

Austin, Charles J., and Stuart Boxerman. *Information Systems for Healthcare Management,* 6th ed. Chicago: Health Administration Press, 2003.

Barry, Robert, Amy C. Murcko, and Clifford E. Brubaker. *The Six Sigma Book for Healthcare.* Chicago: Health Administration Press, 2002.

Bateman, Thomas S., and Carl P. Zeithaml. *Management: Function and Strategy,* 2nd ed. Burr Ridge, Ill.: McGraw-Hill, 1993.

Bayles, Michael D. *Professional Ethics,* 2nd ed. Belmont, Calif.: Wadsworth, 1989.

Beauchamp, Thomas L., and James F. Childress. *Principles of Biomedical Ethics,* 5th ed. New York: Oxford University Press, 2001.

Berkman, Lisa F., and Ichiro Kawachi, eds. *Social Epidemiology.* New York: Oxford University Press, 2000.

Berkowitz, Eric N. *Essentials of Health Care Marketing.* Gaithersburg, Md.: Aspen, 1996.

Berkowitz, Eric N., Louis G. Pol, and Richard K. Thomas. *Healthcare Market Research: Tools and Techniques for Analyzing and Understanding Today's Healthcare Environment.* New York: McGraw-Hill, 1995.

Berlowitz, Dan R., and others. "Quality Improvement Implementation in the Nursing Home," *Health Services Research,* Vol. 38, No. 1 (February 2003): 65–83.

Beyerlein, Michael M., Douglas A. Johnson, and Susan T. Beyerlein, eds. *Team Performance Management: Advances in Interdisciplinary Studies of Work Teams,* Vol. 6. Stamford, Conn.: JAI Press, 2000.

Bickman, Leonard, ed. *Using Program Theory in Evaluation.* New Directions for Program Evaluation Series, No. 33. San Francisco: Jossey-Bass, 1987.

Blake, Robert R., and Anne Adams McCanse. *Leadership Dilemmas–Grid Solutions.* Houston: Gulf, 1991.

Blake, Robert R., and Jane S. Mouton. *The Managerial Grid III: The Key to Leadership Excellence.* Houston: Gulf, 1985.

Bono, Joyce E., and Timothy A. Judge. "Self-Concordance at Work: Toward Understanding the Motivational Effects of Transformational Leaders," *Academy of Management Journal,* Vol. 46, No. 5 (October 2003): 554–571.

Brennan, Troyen A., and others. "Incidence of Adverse Events and Negligence in Hospitalized Patients: Results of the Harvard Medical Practice Study," *New England Journal of Medicine,* Vol. 324, No. 6 (February 7, 1991): 370–376.

Brook, Robert H., and Kathleen N. Lohr. "Efficacy, Effectiveness, Variations and Quality: Boundary-Crossing Research," *Medical Care,* Vol. 23, No. 5 (1985): 710–722.

Brook, Robert H., and Elizabeth A. McGlynn. "Maintaining Quality of Care," in *Health Services Research: Key to Health Policy,* ed. Eli Ginzberg. Cambridge, Mass.: Harvard University Press (1991): 284–314.

Brook, Robert H., Elizabeth A. McGlynn, and Paul G. Shekelle. "Defining and Measuring Quality of Care: A Perspective from U.S. Researchers," *International Journal for Quality in Health Care,* Vol. 12, No. 4 (2000): 281–295.

Burns, James M. *Leadership.* New York: HarperCollins, 1978.

Centers for Disease Control and Prevention. *CDCynergy Content and Framework Workbook.* Atlanta: U.S. Department of Health and Human Services, Office of Communication, Office of the Director, 1999a.

Centers for Disease Control and Prevention. "Framework for Program Evaluation in Public Health," *Morbidity and Mortality Weekly Report,* Vol. 48, No. RR-11 (September 17, 1999b): 1–43.

Charns, Martin P., and Jody Hoffer Gittell. "Work Design," in *Health Care Management: Organization Design and Behavior,* 4th ed., eds. Stephen M. Shortell and Arnold D. Kaluzny. Albany, N.Y.: Delmar Thomson Learning (2000): 191–209.

Chassin, Mark R. "Is Health Care Ready for Six Sigma Quality?" *The Milbank Quarterly,* Vol. 76, No. 4 (1998): 565–591.

Cohen, Susan G., and Diane E. Bailey. "What Makes Teams Work: Group Effectiveness Research from the Shop Floor to the Executive Suite," *Journal of Management,* Vol. 23, No. 3 (1997): 239–290.

Collins, Michelle L. *The Thin Book of 360 Feedback: A Manager's Guide.* Plano, Tex.: Thin Book Company, 2000.

Crosby, Philip B. *Let's Talk Quality.* New York: McGraw-Hill, 1989.

Dansky, Kathryn H., Robert Weech-Maldonado, Gita De Souza, and Janice L. Dreachslin. "Organizational Strategy and Diversity Management: Diversity-Sensitive Orientation as a Moderating Influence," *Health Care Management Review,* Vol. 28, No. 3 (July–September 2003): 243–253.

D'Aunno, Thomas A., Myron D. Fottler, and Stephen J. O'Connor. "Motivating People," in *Health Care Management: Organization Design and Behavior,* 4th ed., eds. Stephen M. Shortell and Arnold D. Kaluzny. Albany, N.Y.: Delmar Thomson Learning (2000): 64–105.

Dean, James W., Jr., and David E. Bowen. "Management Theory and Total Quality: Improving Research and Practice Through Theory Development," *Academy of Management Review,* Vol. 19, No. 3 (July 1994): 392–418.

Delbecq, Andre L., Andrew H. Van de Ven, and David H. Gustafson. *Group Techniques for Program Planning: A Guide to Nominal Group and Delphi Processes.* Mt. Horeb, Wis.: Green Briar, 1986.

Deming, W. Edwards. *Quality, Productivity, and Competitive Position.* Boston: MIT Press, 1982.

Deming, W. Edwards. *Out of the Crisis.* Cambridge, Mass.: Massachusetts Institute of Technology, Center for Advanced Engineering Study, 1986.

Donabedian, Avedis. *Explorations in Quality Assessment and Monitoring, Volume I: The Definition of Quality and Approaches to Its Assessment.* Chicago: Health Administration Press, 1980.

Druskat, Vanessa U., and Jane V. Wheeler. "Managing from the Boundary: The Effective Leadership of Self-Managing Work Teams." *Academy of Management Journal,* Vol. 46, No. 4 (August 2003): 435–457.

DuBrin, Andrew J. *Essentials of Management,* 6th ed. Mason, Ohio: South-Western, 2003.

Erez, Miriam, and Frederick H. Kanfer. "The Role of Goal Acceptance in Goal Setting and Task Performance," *Academy of Management Review* 8 (July 1983): 454–463.

Erez, Miriam P., Christopher Earley, and Charles L. Hulin. "The Impact of Participation on Goal Acceptance and Performance: A Two-Step Model," *Academy of Management Journal* 28 (March 1985): 50–66.

Evans, Robert G., Morris L. Barer, and Theodore R. Marmor, eds. *Why Are Some People Healthy and Others Not? The Determinants of Health of Populations.* New York: Aldine De Gruyter, 1994.

Fayol, Henri. *General and Industrial Management.* Trans. Constance Storrs. London: Sir Isaac Pitman and Sons, 1949.

Fiedler, Fred E. "A Contingency Model of Leadership Effectiveness," in *Advances in Experimental Social Psychology,* ed. Leonard Berkowitz. New York: Academic Press, 1964.

Fiedler, Fred E. *A Theory of Leadership Effectiveness.* New York: McGraw-Hill, 1967.

Filerman, Gary L., and D. David Persaud. "Advocacy," in *Government Relations in the Health Care Industry,* eds. Peggy Leatt and Joseph Mapa. Westport, Conn.: Praeger (2003): 77–93.

Fottler, Myron D. "Strategic Human Resources Management," in *Human Resources in Healthcare: Managing for Success,* eds. Bruce J. Fried and James A. Johnson. Chicago: Health Administration Press (2002): 1–18.

Fottler, Myron D., S. Robert Hernandez, and Charles L. Joiner. *Essentials of Human Resource Management in Health Service Organizations.* Clifton Park, N.Y.: Delmar Learning, 1998.

Frame, J. Davidson. *Managing Projects in Organizations: How to Make the Best Use of Time, Techniques, and People,* 3rd ed. San Francisco: Jossey-Bass, 2003.

French, John R., and Bertram H. Raven. "The Basis of Social Power," in *Studies of Social Power,* ed. Dorwin Cartwright. Ann Arbor, Mich.: Institute for Social Research (1959): 150–167.

Fried, Bruce J., and James A. Johnson, eds. *Human Resources in Healthcare: Managing for Success.* Chicago: Health Administration Press, 2002.

Fried, Bruce J., Sharon Topping, and Thomas G. Rundall. "Groups and Teams in Health Services Organizations," in *Health Care Management: Organizational Design and Behavior,* eds. Stephen M. Shortell and Arnold D. Kaluzny. Albany, N.Y.: Delmar (2000): 154–190.

Gapenski, Louis C. *Healthcare Finance: An Introduction to Accounting and Financial Management,* 2nd ed. Chicago: Health Administration Press, 2002.

Gerteis, Margaret, Susan Edgman-Levitan, Jennifer Daley, and Thomas L. Delbanco, eds. *Through the Patient's Eyes: Understanding and Promoting Patient-Centered Care.* San Francisco: Jossey-Bass, 2002.

Ginter, Peter M., Linda E. Swayne, and W. Jack Duncan. *Strategic Management of Health Care Organizations,* 4th ed. Malden, Mass.: Blackwell Publishing, 2002.

Goleman, Daniel. *Emotional Intelligence.* New York: Bantam Books, 1995.

Goleman, Daniel. "What Makes a Leader?" *Harvard Business Review,* Vol. 76 (November–December 1998): 93–102.

Green, Lawrence W., and Marshall W. Kreuter. *Health Promotion Planning: An Educational and Ecological Approach,* 3rd ed. San Francisco: Mayfield, 1999.

Griffith, John R., and Kenneth R. White. *The Well-Managed Healthcare Organization,* 5th ed. Chicago: Health Administration Press, 2002.

Gulick, Luther, and Lyndall Urwick, eds. *Papers on the Science of Administration.* New York: Institute of Public Administration, 1937.

Hackman, J. Richard. *Leading Teams: Setting the Stage for Great Performance.* Boston: Harvard Business School Press, 2002.

Hage, Jerald. *Theories of Organizations: Forms, Processes, and Transformations.* New York: Wiley-Interscience, 1980.

Ham, Chris, Ruth Kipping, and Hugh McLeod. "Redesigning Work Processes in Health Care: Lessons from the National Health Service," *Milbank Quarterly,* Vol. 81, No. 3 (September 2003): 415–439.

Harris, Dean M. *Contemporary Issues in Healthcare Law and Ethics.* Chicago: Health Administration Press, 2003.

Harris, Thomas E., and John C. Sherblom. *Small Group and Team Communication.* Boston: Allyn & Bacon, 2002.

Health Canada, Social Marketing Network Web site, <http://www.hc-sc.gc.ca/english/socialmarketing>.

Hershey, Paul, and Kenneth H. Blanchard. *Management of Organizational Behavior,* 7th ed. Upper Saddle River, N.J.: Prentice Hall, 1996.

Herzberg, Frederick. "One More Time: How Do You Motivate Employees?" *Harvard Business Review* 87 (September–October 1987): 109–117.

Herzberg, Frederick, Bernard Mausner, and Barbara Snyderman. *The Motivation to Work.* New York: Wiley, 1959.

Hoffman, Douglas K., and John E. G. Bateson. *Essentials of Services Marketing,* 2nd ed. Mason, Ohio: South-Western, 2001.

Holsapple, Clyde W., and Kshiti D. Joshi. "Organizational Knowledge Resources," *Decision Support Systems,* Vol. 31, No. 1 (May 2001): 39–54.

House, Robert J. "A Path-Goal Theory of Leader Effectiveness," *Administrative Science Quarterly* 16 (September 1971): 321–339.

House, Robert J., and Terence R. Mitchell. "Path-Goal Theory of Leadership," *Journal of Contemporary Business* 3 (Autumn 1974): 81–98.

Hudak, Ronald P., Paul P. Brooke Jr., Kenn Finstuen, and James Trounson. "Management Competencies for Medical Practice Executives: Skills, Knowledge, and Abilities Required for the Future," *Journal of Health Administration Education* 15 (Fall 1997): 219–239.

Institute of Medicine. *Medicare: A Strategy for Quality Assurance, Volume I.* Washington, D.C.: National Academy Press, 1990.

Institute of Medicine, National Roundtable on Health Care Quality. *Statement on Quality of Care.* Washington, D.C.:National Academies Press, 1998.

Institute of Medicine, Committee on Quality of Health Care in America. *Crossing the Quality Chasm: A New Health System for the 21st Century.* Washington, D.C.: National Academies Press, 2001.

Intel Corporation. *Intel's Quality System Handbook.* Santa Clara, Calif.: Intel Corporation, <http://developer.intel.com/design/quality/quality.htm>, 2003.

James, Brent C. *Quality Management for Healthcare Delivery.* Chicago: The Health Research and Educational Trust of the American Hospital Association, 1989.

Juran, Joseph M. *Juran on Leadership for Quality: An Executive Handbook.* New York: The Free Press, 1989.

Kass, Nancy E. "An Ethics Framework for Public Health," *American Journal of Public Health,* Vol. 91, No. 11 (November 2001): 1776–1783.

Katz, Daniel, and Robert L. Kahn. "Some Recent Findings in Human Relations Research," in *Readings in Social Psychology,* eds. Guy E. Swanson, Theodore M. Newcomb, and Raymond E. Hartley. New York: Holt, 1952.

Katz, Daniel, and Robert L. Kahn. *The Social Psychology of Organizations.* New York: Wiley, 1978.

Katz, Robert L. "Skills of an Effective Administrator," *Harvard Business Review* 52 (September–October 1974): 90–102.

Kelly, Diane L. *Applying Quality Management in Healthcare.* Chicago: Health Administration Press, 2003.

Kerzner, Harold. *Project Management: A Systems Approach to Planning, Scheduling, and Controlling,* 7th ed. New York: Wiley, 2001.

Keys, Bernard, and Thomas Case. "How to Become an Influential Manager," *The Executive* 4 (November 1990): 38–51.

Kingdon, John W. *Agendas, Alternatives, and Public Policies,* 2nd ed. New York: Harper-Collins, 1995.

Kirkpatrick, Shelly A., and Edwin A. Locke. "Leadership: Do Traits Matter?" *The Executive* 5 (May 1991): 48–60.

Kohn, Linda T., Janet M. Corrigan, and Molla S. Donaldson, eds. *To Err Is Human: Building a Safer Health System.* Washington, D.C.: National Academy Press, 2000.

Kotler, Philip. *Marketing for Non-Profit Organizations,* 2nd ed. Englewood Cliffs, N.J.: Prentice Hall, 1982.

Kotler, Philip. *Marketing Management,* 11th ed. Upper Saddle River, N.J.: Prentice Hall, 2002a.

Kotler, Philip. *Social Marketing,* 2nd ed. Thousand Oaks, Calif.: Sage, 2002b.

Kotler, Philip, and Roberta N. Clarke. *Marketing for Health Care Organizations.* Englewood Cliffs, N.J.: Prentice-Hall, 1987.

Kotler, Philip, and Gerald Zaltman. "Social Marketing: An Approach to Planned Social Change," *Journal of Marketing* 35 (1971): 3–12.

Kotler, Philip, Ned Roberto, and Nancy Lee. *Social Marketing: Improving the Quality of Life,* 2nd ed. Thousand Oaks, Calif.: Sage, 2002.

Kovner, Anthony R., Jeffrey J. Elton, and John Billings. "Transforming Health Management: Evidence-Based Management," *Frontiers of Health Services Management,* Vol. 16, No. 4 (Summer 2000): 3–24.

LaFasto, Frank, and Carl Larson. *When Teams Work Best.* Thousand Oaks, Calif.: Sage, 2001.

Lagarde, François. "Best Practices and Prospects for Social Marketing in Public Health." Speech given at the 89th Annual Conference of the Canadian Public Health Association on Best Practices in Public Health, Montreal, Quebec, June 8, 1998.

Latham, Gary P., and J. James Baldes. "The Practical Significance of Locke's Theory of Goal Setting," *Journal of Applied Psychology* 60 (February 1975): 122–124.

Latham, Gary P., and Edwin A. Locke. "Goal-Setting–A Motivational Technique That Works," in *Motivation and Work Behavior,* 4th ed., eds. Richard M. Steers and Lyman W. Porter. New York: McGraw-Hill (1987): 120–134.

Lepsinger, Richard, and Anntoinette D. Lucia. *The Art and Science of 360° Feedback.* San Francisco: Jossey-Bass, 1997.

Levey, Samuel. "The Leadership Mystique," *Hospital & Health Services Administration* 35 (Winter 1990): 479–480.

Lewin, Kurt. "Frontiers in Group Dynamics: Concept, Method, and Reality in Social Science, Social Equilibria, and Social Change," *Human Relations* 1 (June 1947): 5–41.

Likert, Rensis. *New Patterns of Management.* New York: McGraw-Hill, 1961.

Likert, Rensis. *Past and Future Perspectives on System 4.* Ann Arbor, Mich.: Rensis Likert Associates, 1977.

Litterer, Joseph A. *The Analysis of Organizations.* New York: Wiley, 1965.

Locke, Edwin A. "Toward a Theory of Task Motivation and Incentives," *Organizational Behavior and Performance* 3 (May 1968): 157–189.

Locke, Edwin A. "Purpose Without Consciousness: A Contradiction," *Psychological Reports* 24 (June 1969): 991–1009.

Locke, Edwin A. "The Ubiquity of the Technique of Goal Setting in Theories of and Approaches to Employee Motivation," in *Motivation and Work Behavior,* 4th ed., eds. Richard M. Steers and Lyman W. Porter. New York: McGraw-Hill (1987): 120–134.

Locke, Edwin A., and Gary P. Latham. *A Theory of Goal Setting and Task Performance.* Englewood Cliffs, N.J.: Prentice Hall, 1990.

Longest, Beaufort B., Jr. *Seeking Strategic Advantage Through Health Policy Analysis.* Chicago: Health Administration Press, 1996.

Longest, Beaufort B., Jr., "Managerial Competence at Senior Levels of Integrated Delivery Systems," *Journal of Healthcare Management* 43 (March–April 1998a): 115–135.

Longest, Beaufort B., Jr. "Organizational Change and Innovation," in *Handbook of Health Care Management,* eds. W. Jack Duncan, Peter M. Ginter, and Linda E. Swayne. Malden, Mass.: Blackwell Publishers (1998b): 369–398.

Longest, Beaufort B., Jr., *Health Policymaking in the Untied States,* 3rd ed. Chicago: Health Administration Press, 2002.

Longest, Beaufort B., Jr., Jonathon S. Rakich, and Kurt Darr. *Managing Health Services Organizations and Systems,* 4th ed. Baltimore: Health Professions Press, 2000.

Luallin, Meryl D., and Kevin W. Sullivan, "Marketing in a Changing Environment," in *Ambulatory Care Management,* 3rd ed., eds. Austin Ross, Stephen J. Williams, and Ernest J. Pavlock. Albany, N.Y.: Delmar (1998): 287–307.

Luke, Roice D., Stephen L. Walston, and Patrick Michael Plummer. *Healthcare Strategy: In Pursuit of Competitive Advantage.* Chicago: Health Administration Press, 2004.

Maslow, Abraham H. "A Theory of Human Motivation," *Psychological Review* 50 (July 1943): 370–396.

Maslow, Abraham H. *Eupsychian Management.* Homewood, Ill.: Dorsey-Irwin, 1965.

Maslow, Abraham H. *Motivation and Personality,* 2nd ed. New York: HarperCollins, 1970.

Mathis, Robert L., and John H. Jackson. *Human Resource Management,* 9th ed. Mason, Ohio: South-Western, 2003.

McClelland, David C. *The Achieving Society.* Princeton, N.J.: Van Nostrand, 1961.

McClelland, David C. *Power: The Inner Experience.* New York: Irvington, 1975.

McClelland, David C. *Human Motivation.* Glenview, Ill.: Scott, Foresman, 1985.

McConnell, Charles R. *The Effective Health Care Supervisor,* 5th ed. Gaithersburg, Md.: Aspen Publishers, 2003.

McKenzie, James F., and Jan L. Smeltzer. *Planning, Implementing, and Evaluating Health Promotion Programs: A Primer,* 3rd ed. Boston: Allyn & Bacon, 2001.

McLaughlin, Curtis P., and Arnold D. Kaluzny. "Total Quality Management in Health: Making It Work," *Health Care Management Review,* Vol. 15, No. 3 (Summer 1990): 7–14.

McLaughlin, Curtis P., and Arnold D. Kaluzny. *Continuous Quality Improvement in Health Care: Theory, Implementation and Applications.* Gaithersburg, Md.: Aspen Publishers, 1994.

Mento, Anthony J., Robert P. Steel, and Ronald J. Karren. "A Meta-Analytic Study of the Effects of Goal Setting on Task Performance: 1966–1984," *Organizational Behavior and Human Decision Processes* 39 (February 1987): 52–83.

Miller, Katherine I., and Peter R. Monge. "Participation, Satisfaction, and Productivity: A Meta-Analytic Review," *Academy of Management Journal* 29 (December 1986): 727–753.

Mintzberg, Henry. *The Nature of Managerial Work*. New York: HarperCollins, 1973.

Mintzberg, Henry. "The Manager's Job: Folklore and Fact," *Harvard Business Review* (July–August 1975): 49–61.

Mintzberg, Henry. *The Structuring of Organizations*. Englewood Cliffs, N.J.: Prentice-Hall, 1979.

Mintzberg, Henry. *Structure in Fives: Designing Effective Organizations*. Englewood Cliffs, N.J.: Prentice Hall, 1983.

Mondy, R. Wayne, Robert M. Noe, Shane R. Premeaux, and Judy Bandy Mondy. *Human Resource Management,* 8th ed. Upper Saddle River, N.J.: Prentice Hall, 2002.

Mooney, James D., and Alan C. Reiley. *Onward Industry: The Principles of Organization and Their Significance to Modern Industry*. New York: Harper & Brothers, 1931.

Mowday, Richard T. "Equity Theory Predictions of Behavior in Organizations," in *Motivation and Work Behavior,* 4th ed, eds. Richard M. Steers and Lyman W. Porter. New York: McGraw-Hill (1987): 89–110.

Muchinsky, Paul M. *People at Work: The New Millennium*. Pacific Grove, Calif.: Brooks/Cole, 2000.

Murray, Henry A. *Explorations in Personality*. New York: Oxford University Press, 1938.

National Institute of Standards and Technology. *Healthcare Criteria for Performance Excellence*. Washington, D.C.: National Institute for Standards and Technology, 2003.

Naylor, James C., and Daniel R. Ilgen. "Goal Setting: A Theoretical Analysis of a Motivational Technique," in *Research in Organizational Behavior,* Vol. 6, eds. Barry M. Staw and Larry L. Cummings. Greenwich, Conn.: JAI Press (1984): 95–140.

Neiger, Brad L. *Social Marketing: Making Public Health Sense*. Paper presented at the annual meeting of the Utah Public Health Association. Provo, Utah, 1998.

Nowicki, Michael. *The Financial Management of Hospitals and Healthcare Organizations,* 2nd ed. Chicago: Health Administration Press, 2001.

O'Connor, Stephen J. "Motivating Effective Performance," in *Handbook of Health Care Management,* eds. W. Jack Duncan, Peter M. Ginter, and Linda E. Swayne. Malden, Mass.: Blackwell (1998): 431–470.

Office of Minority Health, U.S. Department of Health and Human Services. *National Standards for Culturally and Linguistically Appropriate Services in Health Care*. Washington, D.C.: U.S. Office of Minority Health, Department of Health and Human Services, March 2001.

Orlikoff, James E., and Mark K. Totten. *The Future of Health Care Governance: Redesigning Boards for a New Era*. Chicago: American Hospital Publishing, 1996.

Page, Ann, ed. *Keeping Patients Safe: Transforming the Work Environment of Nurses*. Washington, D.C.: National Academies Press, 2004.

Parasuraman, A., Valaries A. Zeithaml, and Leonard L. Berry. "SERVQUAL: A Multiple Item Scale for Measuring Consumer Perceptions of Service Quality." *Journal of Retailing,* Vol. 64, No. 1 (Spring 1988): 12–40.

Patient Self-Determination Act (Public Law 101-508).

Patton, Michael Q. *Utilization-Focused Evaluation: The New Century Text*. Thousand Oaks, Calif.: Sage, 1997.

Peters, Lawrence H., Darnell D. Hartke, and John T. Pohlman. "Fiedler's Contingency Theory of Leadership: An Application of the Meta-Analysis Procedures of Schmidt and Hunter," *Psychological Bulletin* 97 (March 1985): 274–285.

Petersen, Donna J., and Greg R. Alexander. *Needs Assessment in Public Health: A Practical Guide for Students and Professionals.* New York: Kluwer Academic/Plenum Publishers, 2001.

Pettigrew, Andrew M., Richard W. Woodman, and Kim S. Cameron. "Studying Organizational Change and Development: Challenges for Future Research," *Academy of Management Journal,* Vol. 44, No. 4 (August 2001): 697–713.

Pointer, Dennis D., and Julianne P. Sanchez. "Leadership: A Framework for Thinking and Acting," in *Health Care Management: Organization Design and Behavior,* eds. Stephen M. Shortell and Arnold D. Kaluzny. Albany, N.Y.: Delmar (2000): 106–129.

Project Management Institute. *A Guide to the Project Management Body of Knowledge.* Newton Square, Pa.: Project Management Institute, 2000.

Rawls, John. *A Theory of Justice,* revised. Cambridge, Mass.: Harvard University Press, 1999.

Renger, Ralph, and Allison Titcomb. "A Three-Step Approach to Teaching Logic Models," *American Journal of Evaluation* 23 (Winter 2002): 493–503.

Revere, Lee, and Ken Black. "Integrating Six Sigma with Total Quality Management: A Case Example for Measuring Medication Errors," *Journal of Healthcare Management,* Vol. 48, No. 6 (November–December 2003): 377–391.

Rice, James A. *Leadership Insights.* La Jolla, Calif.: The International Health Summit, 2003.

Robbins, Stephen P., and Mary K. Coulter. *Management,* 8th ed. Upper Saddle River, N.J.: Prentice Hall, 2004.

Ross, Austin, Frederick J. Wenzel, and Joseph W. Mitlyng. *Leadership for the Future: Core Competencies in Healthcare.* Chicago: Health Administration Press, 2002.

Ross, Helen S., and Paul R. Mico. *Theory and Practice in Health Education.* San Francisco: Mayfield, 1980.

Rossi, Peter H., Mark W. Lipsey, and Howard E. Freeman. *Evaluation: A Systematic Approach,* 7th ed. Thousand Oaks, Calif.: Sage, 2003.

Schwartz, Robert H. "Coping with Unbalanced Information About Decision-Making Influence for Nurses," *Hospital & Health Services Administration* 35 (Winter 1990): 547–559.

Schwarz, Miriam, Suzanne E. Landis, and John E. Rowe. "A Team Approach to Quality Improvement," *Family Practice Management,* Vol. 6, No. 4 (April 1999): 25–33.

Seglin, Jeffrey L. "Ethics: Good for Goodness' Sake," *CFO Magazine* (October 2002): 76.

Senge, Peter M. *The Fifth Discipline: The Art and Practice of the Learning Organization.* New York: Bantam Books, 1990.

Simon, Herbert A. *Models of Bounded Rationality.* Cambridge, Mass.: MIT Press, 1982.

Simons-Morton, Bruce G., Walter H. Greene, and Nell H. Gottlieb. *Introduction to Health Education and Health Promotion,* 2nd ed. Prospect Heights, Ill.: Waveland Press, 1995.

Smith, William A. "Social Marketing: An Evolving Definition," *American Journal of Health Behavior,* Vol. 24, No. 1 (January–February 2000): 11–17.

Spear, Steven, and H. Kent Bowen. "Decoding the DNA of the Toyota Production System," *Harvard Business Review,* Vol. 77, No. 5 (September–October 1999): 96–106.

Steers, Richard M., and Lyman W. Porter, *Motivation and Leadership at Work.* 4th ed. New York: McGraw-Hill (1987): 111–120.

Stogdill, Ralph M. "Personal Factors Associated with Leadership," *Journal of Psychology* 25 (January 1948): 35–71.

Stogdill, Ralph M. *Handbook of Leadership: A Survey of the Literature.* New York: Free Press, 1974.

Stogdill, Ralph M., and Alvin E. Coons, eds. *Leadership Behavior: Its Description and Measurement.* Research Monograph No. 88. Columbus: Bureau of Business Research, Ohio State University, 1957.

Tannenbaum, Robert, and Warren H. Schmidt. "How to Choose a Leadership Pattern," *Harvard Business Review* 51 (May–June 1973): 162–180.

Thompson, James D. *Organizations in Action.* New York: McGraw-Hill, 1967.

Timmreck, Thomas C. *Planning, Program Development, and Evaluation: A Handbook for Health Promotion, Aging, and Health Services.* Boston: Jones and Bartlett, 1995.

Toegel, Ginka, and Jay A. Conger. "360-Degree Assessment: Time for Reinvention," *Academy of Management Learning and Education,* Vol. 2, No. 3 (September 2003): 297–311.

Tuckman, Bruce W., and Mary Ann C. Jensen. "Stages of Small-Group Development Revisited," *Group and Organizational Studies* 2 (Summer 1977): 419–427.

U.S. General Accounting Office. *Management Practices: U.S. Companies Improve Performance Through Quality Efforts.* GAO/NSIAD-91-190. Washington, D.C.: U.S. General Accounting Office, 1991.

Van Fleet, David D., and Gary A. Yukl. "A Century of Leadership Research," in *Contemporary Issues in Leadership,* 3rd ed., eds. William E. Rosenbach and Robert L. Taylor. Boulder, Colo.: Westview Press (1989): 65–90.

Vroom, Victor H. *Work and Motivation.* New York: Wiley, 1964.

Vroom, Victor H. "A New Look at Managerial Decision Making," *Organizational Dynamics,* Vol. 1, No. 4 (Spring 1973): 66-80.

Vroom, Victor H., and Arthur G. Jago. *The New Leadership: Managing Participation in Organizations.* Upper Saddle River, N.J.: Prentice Hall, 1988.

Vroom, Victor H., and Philip W. Yetton. *Leadership and Decision Making.* Pittsburgh: University of Pittsburgh Press, 1973.

W. K. Kellogg Foundation. *Logic Model Development Guide.* Battle Creek, Mich.: W. K. Kellogg Foundation, <www.wkkf.org>, 2001.

Walshe, Kieran, and Thomas G. Rundall. "Evidence-Based Management: From Theory to Practice in Health Care," *The Milbank Quarterly,* Vol. 79, No. 3 (September 2001): 429–457.

Walster, Elaine H., G. William Walster, and Ellen Berscheid. *Equity: Theory and Research.* Boston: Allyn & Bacon, 1978.

Weber, Max. *The Theory of Social and Economic Organization.* Trans. A. M. Henderson and Talcott Parsons. New York: The Free Press, 1947.

Weiss, Carol H. *Evaluation: Methods for Studying Programs and Policies,* 2nd ed. Upper Saddle River, N.J.: Prentice Hall, 1998.

Wood, Robert E., and Edwin A. Locke. "Goal Setting and Strategy Effects on Complex Tasks," in *A Theory of Goal Setting and Task Performance,* eds. Edwin A. Locke and Gary P. Latham. Englewood Cliffs, N.J.: Prentice Hall (1990): 293–319.

World Health Organization. Preamble to the Constitution of the World Health Organization as adopted by the International Health Conference, New York, June 12–22, 1946; signed on July 22, 1946, by the representatives of sixty-one states (Official Records of the World Health Organization, no. 2, p. 100) and entered into force on April 7, 1948.

Yukl, Gary A. *Leadership in Organizations,* 5th ed. Upper Saddle River, N.J.: Prentice Hall, 2002.

Zuckerman, Howard S., and William L. Dowling. "The Managerial Role," in *Essentials of Health Care Management,* eds. Stephen M. Shortell and Arnold D. Kaluzny. Albany, N.Y.: Delmar Publishers (1997): 34–62.

INDEX